PRAISE FOR

Energy Wellness for

"Cyndi has a real gift and has put her heart and soul into *Energy Wellness for Your Pet*—a book the world needs now more than ever. Her goal is the same as mine: to prevent suffering and do no harm."—Dr. Stephen R. Blake, DVM, CVA, CVH, Usui Reiki Master Shaman

"[Cyndi's] guidance will bring about enhanced health, happiness, and bonding for you and your animal companions—furred, feathered, and invertebrates. Bravo, Cyndi!"—Joan Ranquet, animal communicator, healer, author, and founder of Communication with All Life University

"A well-written, inspiring look into the subtle energies of our pets and how we can work with this energy to understand our animal friends…Cyndi speaks from the heart and shares personal stories that teach through example and will deeply affect you. I honestly couldn't put this book down…A must-read for anyone who has a pet."—Melissa Alvarez, author of *Animal Frequency* and *Llewellyn's Little Book of Spirit Animals*

"Cyndi Dale's brilliant book expertly teaches readers how to apply energetic concepts and techniques to improve a pet's emotional, physical, and spiritual well-being…Highly recommended for all animal lovers!"—Madisyn Taylor, cofounder of *DailyOM*

Energy Wellness
for your Pet

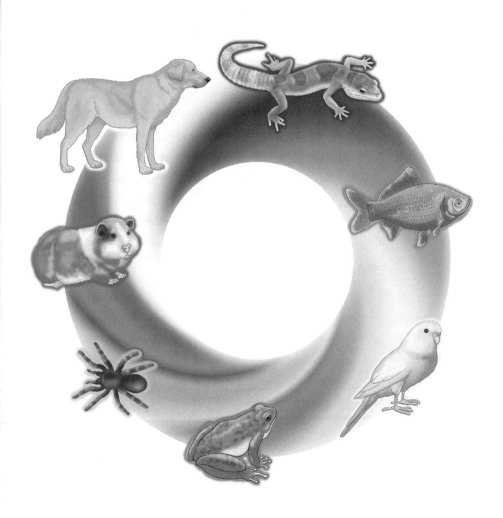

About Cyndi Dale

Cyndi Dale (Minneapolis, MN), pictured on the cover with her dogs Honey and Lucky, is an internationally renowned author, speaker, healer, and business consultant. She is president of Life Systems Services, through which she has conducted over 65,000 client sessions and presented training classes throughout Europe, Asia, and the Americas. Visit her online at Cyndidale.com.

Energy Wellness
for your Pet

**A Subtle Energy Companion for
Better Bonding, Health & Happiness**

Cyndi Dale

Llewellyn Publications
WOODBURY, MINNESOTA

FIRST EDITION
First Printing, 2019

Book design and edit by Rebecca Zins
Cover design by Shira Atakpu
Cover photo by Katie Cannon Photography
Illustrations by Mary Ann Zapalac

Llewellyn Publications is a registered trademark of Llewellyn Worldwide Ltd.

Library of Congress Cataloging-in-Publication Data
Names: Dale, Cyndi, author.
Title: Energy wellness for your pet : a subtle energy companion for better
 bonding, health, and happiness / Cyndi Dale.
Description: First edition. | Woodbury, Minnesota : Llewellyn Publications,
 2019. | Includes bibliographical references and index.
Identifiers: LCCN 2018046650 (print) | LCCN 2018048339 (ebook) | ISBN
 9780738758497 (ebook) | ISBN 9780738758435 (alk. paper)
Subjects: LCSH: Alternative veterinary medicine.
Classification: LCC SF745.5 (ebook) | LCC SF745.5 .D35 2019 (print) | DDC
 636.089/55—dc23
LC record available at https://lccn.loc.gov/2018046650

Llewellyn Publications
A Division of Llewellyn Worldwide Ltd.
2143 Wooddale Drive
Woodbury, MN 55125-2989

www.llewellyn.com

Printed in the United States of America

Contents

Chapter One
Explaining the Unexplainable Bond   9

Chapter Two
Your Pet's Personal Energetic Signature   31

Chapter Six

Energetic Solutions That Create More Well-Being   143

Chapter Seven

Vibrational Medicines and Tools for Health and Well-Being   167

Chapter Eight
Of Dying, Death, and the Afterlife 193

Exercises and Tips

Illustrations

Charts

Disclaimer

The information in this book is not intended to be used to diagnose or treat a medical, emotional, or behavioral condition for either pets or humans. To address medical, behavioral, or therapeutic issues, please consult a licensed professional; for pets, these are most frequently available through licensed veterinarian services.

The author and publisher are not responsible for any conditions that require a licensed professional, and we encourage you to consult a professional if you have any questions about the use or efficacy of the techniques or insights in this book. References in this book are given for informational purposes alone and do not constitute an endorsement.

All case studies and descriptions of persons have been changed or altered so as to be unrecognizable. Any likeness to actual persons living or dead is strictly coincidental.

Introduction

*Perhaps the greatest gift an
animal has to offer is a permanent
reminder of who we really are.*

Nick Trout, *Love Is the Best Medicine*

The young man could hardly hold on to the struggling puppy. Finally, a young woman emerged from the café, which was named Captain's. She laughed and reached for the tiny Labrador.

I was startled. The previous night I had dreamed about a baby Labrador with a bright purple collar, upon which was inscribed a single word: "Captain's." I groaned. It looked like I was being directed to get a new puppy. All that was missing in the scene was the collar.

Let me explain.

My son and I were in northern Minnesota on vacation. We had left our two dogs back at the cabin while we hunted for breakfast. One of our dogs was aging, and my son and I had discussed looking for a "replacement" puppy—sometime in the future. Then I had my dream, which seemed to have been both a premonition and a directive. The young couple, having just picked up their new puppy, were happy to give us directions to "The Captain's Labradors."

Within the hour, my son and I were snuggling with armfuls of wiggly puppies. Guess which one we picked? The yellow Lab wearing a thin purple tie. Its mom had picked up the chubby babe in her mouth and plopped it in my son's lap.

1

"That's Mr. Purple," the breeder said, having obviously named the puppy after the color of its collar. "He's the first to the food bowl and wags his tail the most often." Though we renamed the puppy "Lucky," I still have the purple collar in a scrapbook.

We all love our pets, and not only the ever-popular dog or cat. I'll never forget my pet turtle named Wilma, who grew to enormous proportions. When she couldn't maneuver in her tank anymore, I let her trudge around the house for exercise.

One morning, Wilma plunked down near a sack and wouldn't budge. Curious, I opened the bag. There was my son's school essay! He had searched in vain for it that morning before I had to rush him to school without it. Thanks to Wilma, I could drop off the essay before it was due. Wilma had saved the day.

Lucky and Wilma are special. The same is true of every pet, no matter which of the seven pet families they hail from: mammal, rodent, avian, reptile, arthropod, amphibian, and aquatic. There are many reasons that each pet is so extraordinary, and we'll explore dozens of them in this book. Crucial to these discussions is one central tenet, however, which is that pets are spiritual beings. As such, they have a soul, which incarnates in order to learn critical lessons about concepts like love and purpose. The pet/human bond is a vital part of a pet's wisdom-gathering. And guess what? The living beings that share this planet with us are often our most notable teachers.

This statement is true of the members of all seven pet families, no matter if they are wild or domesticated. It's also true of the various types of domesticated natural beings, which are further defined as companions, livestock, or working animals. I believe that all of our natural friends have souls, but their purposes, in relation to humans, are different. I'll further explore these distinctions in chapter 1. For now, know that this book is primarily devoted to the souls that incarnate as domestic companions, or pets.

Why does a pet's soul become a pet and not a person? For what reason might it become a bird, a cat, or a frog, rather than a different type of natural being? In this book we'll look at issues like these and so many more, including the ways that a pet processes *karma*, its personal history, and serves *dharma*, a higher purpose. We'll examine the exact nature of the pet/human bond and the hidden causes of a pet's behavioral, psychological, physical, and spiritual challenges.

Through these and other discussions, you'll learn how to assist your pets no matter what they're going through, and subsequently become more of your "true self" in the process. This journey is only possible because we're undertaking it through the most universal lens of all: energy.

Everything is made of energy, which is information that moves. There are two types of energy, however, and understanding the differences between them is critical to making use of this book—and loving your pet in the best possible way. In a nutshell, there are physical and subtle energies.

Most pet books present ways to understand and care for your pet through the viewpoint of physical energy. Physical energy is measurable. It is rock-solid and constitutes what we know through our five senses. If your pet is sick, a physically oriented book might outline disease symptoms and advocate useful medicines. If the pet is a persnickety eater, the book will suggest delectable recipes. While these and other allopathic procedures are vital, they are somewhat limited. You see, physical reality—including a pet's problem—often begins in the "other" world of subtle energy.

Also called mystical, psychic, spiritual, and quantum energy, subtle energy actually runs the material world, forming the latticework that organizes physical energies. Subtle energies make up the substance of a pet's soul, help determine the pet's genetic programming, and determine which human companion a pet will be attracted to. Subtle energies decide which foods might be nourishing or not, how a pet might respond to a crisis, and which psychological factors could attract specific microbial vulnerabilities. Subtle energies even explain the "Lucky dream" I described, which led me to purchasing my favorite yellow Labrador! You see, nearly anything that happens to a pet is initiated by the actions of subtle energies. This means that the pet owner who yearns to make a real difference in their pet's life has to know how to analyze and direct subtle energies.

I should know. I've been employing subtle energy knowledge for decades. In fact, I'm quite an expert on the topic of subtle energy, having written nearly twenty-five books about energetic matters. Through my interactions with over 65,000 human clients, I've also assisted thousands with their pets. And, as you have already surmised, I've utilized subtle data to tend to my own pets.

As a case in point, while raising two children (and a foster daughter, for a while) as a single mother, I also provided a home for two dogs, a cat, two turtles, and a guinea pig. I absolutely had to take all my energy concepts and techniques to heart when the entourage expanded to include several fish, two frogs, and a bunny rabbit. The humans in the zoo were greatly outnumbered. You can only imagine the multiple needs and crises that needed constant management, from illnesses to the chasing of the cat by the dogs and rabbit. I employed the same ideas that you'll learn in this book to create a loving, healthy, and amusing ecosystem. Every pet met its utmost potential, sometimes literally. For instance, Max, the guinea pig, didn't pass until he was nine years old, although the average age of most guinea pigs is four years old. (The clear leader of the pack, Max *had* to stay around.)

So you can apply subtle energy knowledge and tools to your own pet care, I've summarized the most vital data in this book. First, I'll educate you about energy—specifically, the two different types of energy. You'll also learn about the two different bodily systems that govern your pet's energies. In living beings, subtle energies are managed by the subtle energetic anatomy, which is composed of subtle centers, channels, and fields. In turn, these subtle structures regulate the physical organs, tissues, and fields. Of the subtle structures, the most imperative to understand are the twelve chakras, subtle energy centers that administer all physical, psychological, and spiritual functions in living beings, including pets.

Some of you might ask, "Why twelve chakras? I thought there were only seven!" There are actually multiple chakra systems used by different cultures around the world that feature between three and dozens of chakras. Although most esoteric books showcase only the seven in-body chakras, I find that knowledge of the additional five out-of-body chakras is critical to making a true difference in a pet's life. Knowledge of these extra-special chakras will greatly contribute to your ability to assess a pet's issues and arrive at powerful subtle solutions.

Most importantly, I'll show you how to apply knowledge about these chakras, as well as their related fields, to perform everything from figuring out the reason a pet is sick or behaving badly to clearing an emotional trauma. This education will also serve as the basis for deciphering your pet's personal "energetic signature," or the code that makes them unique; intuitively communicating with your pet; and unearthing your pet's past lives. And we'll stretch this data even further. You'll also be taught how to assess and clean the energies between you and your pet, release negative entities, and select vibrational medicines, such as flower essences and essential oils, to bolster your pet's health and well-being—and so much more.

Throughout this book you'll frequently employ my two signature practices, which I present in many of my books. Called Spirit-to-Spirit and Healing Streams of Grace, these processes will help you become a near-instant energy professional. If you already know these techniques, you'll love relating them to pet care. If they are new to you, you'll be thrilled at how easy they are to use. I predict that you'll apply them in nearly every pet endeavor.

Since a good map makes all journeys easier, here are the book's eight chapters with the theme of each summarized in a single phrase.

> **Chapter 1, The Bond:** Presents the story of how a pet's soul moves across time, from past lives to the human home to the afterlife. I'll explore this journey through the lenses of karma, dharma, and energy, explaining the various roles played by the physical and subtle energy systems. I'll also briefly examine the basic differences in purpose between domesticated and wild natural (animal, bird, etc.) souls.

> **Chapter 2, The Signature:** Pet groups, species, and individual souls are imprinted with energetic codes that convey meaning. These add up to an overarching energetic signature that describes your pet.
>
> In this chapter you'll first learn the codes for the seven groupings and the individual species we'll be covering in this book. These are as follows:

> > *Mammals:* dogs, cats, horses, rabbits, ferrets, and pigs
> >
> > *Rodents:* gerbils, hamsters, chinchillas, guinea pigs, fancy rats, and mice
> >
> > *Birds:* parakeets, parrots, canaries, macaws, and domesticated chickens, turkeys, doves, pigeons, ducks, and geese
> >
> > *Reptiles:* snakes, lizards, iguanas, and turtles

Arthropods: spiders, such as tarantulas; crabs, regular
and hermit; ants, caterpillars, and centipedes

Amphibians: frogs, newts, salamanders, and toads

Aquatic: fish, fresh and salt water, including angelfish,
goldfish, rainbow fish, koi, and guppies

You'll discover how your pet's particular history and personality fit into the picture and apply the Spirit-to-Spirit process to formulate your pet's personal energetic signature. This insight will help you focus on your pet's specific needs when performing an energy analysis and healing.

Chapter 3, The Subtle Energy System: After examining the benefits of working with the subtle energy anatomy, which includes subtle centers, channels, and fields, we'll get down to business and focus on the chakras. Each of the chakras in my twelve-chakra system governs specific physical, psychological, and spiritual functions. No matter which type of pet you have, the chapter's illustrations will help you locate your pet's chakras.

Chapter 4, Pet Communication: How do you comprehend what's happening inside of your pet? How can you best send a message to your pet or connect with their spiritual guide? I'll present four chakra-based styles, as well as an all-inclusive mystical style, for intuitive pet communication.

Chapter 5, Energetic Issues: Many issues reduce to a subtle energy imbalance. In this chapter you'll first learn about trauma, the underlying cause of most pet problems. There are various types of traumas, however, and we'll cover the major ones, including energetic absorption, soul possession, emotional challenges, and microbial infections. Included in this chapter is a chart that will enable you to assess a pet's presenting physical, psychological, behavioral, and spiritual-based problems as they relate to the chakras. This chart will serve as an invaluable long-term resource, as you'll be able to refer to it whenever your pet exhibits stress or difficulties.

Chapter 6, Energetic Solutions: It's time to create more well-being and happiness for your pet and your pet/human relationship. This in-depth chapter will reveal ways to formulate solutions for all pet-related challenges based on an energetic analysis. I'll also take you on a quick trip through the chakras, sharing tips for working generically with each chakra and specifically their main organs and bodily parts. You'll be able to return to this list when issues arise with your pet.

Chapter 7, Vibrational Tools: The subtle energy aficionado can employ any number of energetic tools to support their pet's development. In this chapter we'll explore vibrational medicines, including the use of touch, color, stone therapy, toning, and essential oils.

Chapter 8, (Happy) Endings: How can you assist a pet—and yourself—through the pet's dying process? How might you aid one pet with the loss of another one? Are there ways to encourage afterlife contact between you and a pet's soul? All pet/human relationships end at death—or do they? This chapter will help you complete the circle that began when your pet entered your life, whichever lifetime that might have been, and keep it going beyond the earth plane.

As you'll discover, learning "all things energy" about your pet and your pet-human relationship will do more than improve matters for all concerned. It will awaken you to love, for love is the ultimate goal of any pet/human dance and is truly the essence of all that is.

Chapter One
Explaining the
Unexplainable Bond

They are not brethren, they are not
underlings; they are other Nations,
caught with ourselves in the net of
life and time, fellow prisoners of the
splendor and travail of the earth.

Henry Beston

Most of us would say that our pets mean everything to us. The opposite is true as well: we are our pet's entire world. What exactly makes this seemingly unexplainable bond so significant?

To respond to this question, this chapter starts with a journey. Together, we will visit the "First Age," a Hopi term for the beginning of Creation. During that time period, the human nation lived peacefully with nonhuman nations, including the animals, birds, and reptiles. The connection you feel with your pet is an echo of this original bond.

This historical review will lead into a thorough conversation about the contemporary blessings exchanged through the pet/human relationship, and then an exploration of how—and why—a pet enters our life. To help explain these concepts, I'll showcase a story. This tale will reveal how a single pet soul traverses across time and also help me define important terms, such as spirit, soul, mind, body, karma, and dharma. Next, we'll drop squarely into the book's theme: energetics.

In order to truly understand and support your pets, and also enhance your relationship with them, you must have a decent understanding of energy.

Everything is made of energy. There are, however, two types of energy, which are physical and subtle. Comprehending the major differences between these energies, as well as the anatomies that manage each, is the key to enjoying a happy, healthy pet and pet/human relationship. It's also the only way to make tangible the echoes of love that still link the human and nonhuman nations.

And now we're going to explore the ever-evolving and amazing pet/human bond that began ever so long ago.

The First Age
When the Nations Shared Their Wisdom

As stated, there is a reason for the inexplicable and wondrous bond between pets and humans. The explanation relies on a brief historical lesson.

According to the Hopi, the earth has undergone several destructions and rebirths; in fact, we are currently living in the fourth start-up, called the Fourth Age. The Hopis aren't the only culture that believe the same. Societies including the Hindu, Greek, Mayan, Zuni, Navajo, Egyptian, Persian, Aztec, Cherokee, Sumerian, Celt, and Norse have also acknowledged this death-and-rebirth cycle, whether they employ the term "age," "epoch," or "world." What all descriptions have in common is the idea that during the First Age, humans and other natural beings lived in concert.

According to the Hopi, the plants, animals, birds, and other nonhuman nations were actually created before the human nation. These natural beings were well loved by the Mother and Father Creator, as "all the power of creation flowed through them" (Waters 1963, 6). Humans, created next, were meant to occupy a different but equally special place in creation. We were to employ the Creator's wisdom, increasing in knowledge while living peacefully with the nonhuman nations. What humans knew then, which we don't remember now, is that all nations were considered part of the same earthly family and were required to care for each other.

In order to assure connectivity, all living beings were equipped with the same subtle energy organs as existed in the physical earth itself—in other words, the chakras, the Hindu word describing the subtle energy centers that regulate all aspects of life. Chakras will be a major focus of this book. In fact, you'll employ chakra knowledge to accomplish everything from analyzing a pet's problems to creating elegant solutions. The ancient Hopi worked with five essential subtle centers. These were the kopavi, the spiritual doorway at the crown, which accesses energy from the Creator; the forehead center, which enables everyone to think for themselves; the throat center, which vibrates with earthly knowledge; the heart center, which discerns between good and evil; and the solar plexus center, which manages life functions. The Hopi knew that as long as these energy centers were aligned within a living being, there would be no illness. The chakras were therefore considered a sort of "divine blueprint" that kept the earth and all living beings safe, healthy, and interconnected.

And then humans started disconnecting from their subtle centers.

According to the Hopi, a manipulative being convinced people that they were better than animals and didn't need to tap into the spiritual wisdom of their chakras nor heed their nonhuman friends. Humans started treating their nonhuman friends cruelly, causing them to draw away. Confused, natural beings became wild, and chaos ensued. The resulting evil brought about the end of the First Age.

A few humans managed to retain the Creator's wisdom in between the First and Second Ages. Rising from the ashes, these people accessed their subtle centers to make wise decisions and bond with nonhuman beings. The centers served to direct-connect them to both the earth and the Creator. But once again, violence and greed took over. People again separated from the nonhuman nations and dissociated from their sacred energy centers. Since then, the Second and Third Ages have also fallen, and our Fourth Age isn't looking so good (Waters 1963, 6–15).

The only way to stop or delay the destruction of the current age, according to Hopi elders, is to return the world to its first order. To accomplish this, we humans must live again in harmony with the nonhuman nations (Waters 1963, 182). How best to do this but to better our relationship with our pets? Our pets can restore us, even as we restore them, to the love that echoes in our hearts.

Other cultures also attribute great significance to the early relationship between the nonhuman and human families. In fact, the nonhuman nations sometimes come out ahead on the intelligence scale. For instance, the Creek Indians believe that early humans were so dim-witted and selfish that they couldn't even recognize the Creator's first instructions. These instructions were directives for living a life replete with purpose and meaning. Concerned, the Creator hid knowledge about these instructions in animal and plant creatures, trying to force humans to seek assistance from beings they assumed were less noteworthy. Because of pride, humans wouldn't stoop so low. Subsequently, we are missing out on the secrets of the universe, along with the aid, knowledge, blessings, and other gifts our nonhuman friends can provide (Grantham 2002, 255).

The members of all nonhuman nations offer unique wisdom to each other and also to humans. For the purpose of understanding the significance of your personal pet relationships, it's important to more pointedly define what I mean by the term *pet*. After all, members of the seven categories of families featured in this book—mammals, rodents, birds, reptiles, arthropods, amphibians, and aquatic fish—can exist in wild and domesticated states. In addition, there are several types of domesticated natural beings. Which type do I mean when I use the word *pet*? Let's briefly examine this question from practical and energetic perspectives.

Wild versus Domestic Beings
The Main Differences

From a normative point of view, the natural beings in every one of the seven categories we're discussing in this book, as well as other types of animals, birds, and the like, are labeled as either wild or domesticated. It's vital to understand the differences between these two groupings—and to further break down the domestic category—to know what a pet is and to fully embrace the amazing importance of the pet/human relationship.

In general, wild beings naturally live independently from people. Domesticated beings rely upon humans for their well-being and interact closely with them on a daily basis. This isn't a hard-core definition. Imagine that a family moves out of their neighborhood and leaves their cat behind. That cat might now become wild, in which case it's called "feral." While it doesn't rely fully on humans to survive, the cat might still relate to them. Maybe one neighbor puts out a food bowl every so often and another keeps the shed door open during storms.

On the other side of the coin, some natural beings begin their lives as wild but become domesticated. A sampling includes orphaned wolves, captured monkeys, elephants reared by people, and animals in breeding programs. Exotics are a specific sort of wild creature. These unusual natural beings, such as striped skunks, lions, alligators, pythons, and more, are usually forced into captivity and treated as domestic. They might fraternize with humans but never truly adapt to domestication.

Just as there are distinctions amongst wild beings, so are there differences between domesticated beings. The three main types of domesticated natural beings are working animals, livestock, and companion pets. Farm horses and mules are examples of working animals. Cows, sheep, and goats qualify as livestock. As important as these types of natural beings are, by and large, this book is focused on companion pets—and their souls—because these are the beings that interact with us on every level of consciousness: physical, psychological, spiritual, and energetic.

In comparison to wild natural beings, a companion pet is dependent on us physically. As we'll examine in the next section, sometimes companion pets return the favor. Psychologically, we affect the companion pet's emotional health and vice versa. Spiritually, our soul is often bonded with a pet's soul, karmically or dharmically; not only that, we often exchange psychic messages. Energetically, our chakras constantly interrelate with those of a pet, sharing information, support, and sometimes even illnesses, memories, and issues. We'll explore all of these ideas in this book.

In comparison, wild animals usually show up in our life accidentally or to assist with delivering an omen or message. We'll further explore this latter concept in chapter 2. Our relationship with working animals and livestock is typically limited to physical collaborations, including the exchange of energy between physically oriented chakras. It's infrequent to interact psychologically or spiritually with these types of domesticated beings. Of course, a farm horse can become a companion pet if the relationship moves beyond mere physical components; same with that of a special goat or sheep. Overall, however, the pet companions that occupy our hearts are the most apt to help us fulfill the human-to-nonhuman pledge that endures from the First Age. Because of that, this book is devoted to the companions that teach, lead, and heal—those we call our "pets."

Might our companion pets actually hold the wisdom that we are collectively and individually seeking? If dozens of creation myths are to be believed, the answer is yes. The question is, are we ready to listen?

The Gifts Given by Our Pets

How often do you really listen to your pet or know what blessings they might be offering? It's not always easy to discern the messages and gifts they bring us, as a friend of mine recently learned.

Molly was concerned about her cat. No matter how much she fed him, Felix would meow and scratch at the lower kitchen cupboard near the oven, where she stored his food. Even after he was fed, Felix would return to his position at the cupboard and start protesting all over again.

Molly called and asked if I could figure out what was up with Felix. Did she need to bring him to a vet? Were there mice dancing in the cupboard? I only received a single intuitive flash: the smell of a sickly aroma. I suggested that Molly bring Felix to the vet but also call in a technician to check out the toxic odor.

A few days later, Molly called me back. "There was a gas leak from the oven on the other side of the cupboard," she said, shocked. "I guess my cat was warning me."

Had Felix physically smelled the gas leak? Had his psychic senses given the red alert? Pets have intuitive abilities that can far outshine our own. In any case, once the technician fixed the leak, Felix returned to his normal and fairly lazy state.

This story is only one of thousands I've heard about the uncanny blessings provided humans by their pets. Some of the gifts they grant are physical. Others are more mysterious, qualifying as psychological or spiritual. Either way, it seems that our ancestors were right: our pets display attributes that humans do not.

Take the common household cat. Did you know that a house cat's purr improves bone density and promotes healing, not only within the bones, but also in tendons and ligaments (Lyons 2003)? Proof perfect is the fact that cats don't incur bone disease, except where the vibrational intensity of the purr is the weakest, which is at their paws (Peterson, n.d.).

How about that pet dog? A dog's saliva contains proteins that heal wounds twice as fast than if the injury is left alone (Goodnet 2015). And pets including cats, rabbits, and guinea pigs raise immunities and decrease the numbers of colds and ear infections in children (Rovner 2012). But you don't have to own the proverbial dog, cat, rabbit, or rodent to benefit from pet companionship. Owning any pet seems to do the job.

Case in point: studies reveal that pet owners complain of fewer physical ailments, such as headaches and hay fever, than do non-pet owners. Whether the pet is friendly Fido or sneaky Snake, its presence can reduce cholesterol, triglyceride levels, and hypertension. Having a pet also manufactures smiles, increasing the overall happiness in people of all ages (Pet Health Council, n.d.).

Pets can also be lifesavers, alerting people to healthcare crises. Consider dogs. Equipped with about 220 million scent receptors—as compared to our five million—they can sniff out tiny changes in human chemistry. For example, they can smell the presence of cancer cells, detect an upcoming narcolepsy fit, perceive an emerging migraine, sense a blood sugar dip in diabetics, and predict a seizure (Heimbuch 2016).

So far, all the examples I've provided illustrate a few of the many documented physical and psychological benefits imparted by our pets. But given that they are spiritual beings, pets also contribute spiritual gains. I'll give you a real-life client example.

My client Gertrude's best friend was Rosy, a Chilean rose hair tarantula. These are gentle beings. Although frightening to look at, they are about as speedy as a rock. Rosy physically dwelled in an aquarium, but her soul wandered at night, often straight into Gertrude's dreams.

As you'll discover in chapter 2, all species function on a specific set of codes. Spiders exhibit maternal traits; they can also reveal what to retain or keep out of the web of our lives. In particular, Rosy could sense who was trustworthy or not, as proven one night in Gertrude's dreams. That night, Rosy appeared in clear view, her hairy arms casting dark shadows over an image of Gertrude's newly minted boyfriend. Based on Rosy's message, Gertrude ran a deeper background check on the man and discovered that he was married.

Pets certainly improve our lives, but they also need us to return the favor.

The Gifts We Owe Our Pets

Love is a two-way street. Our pets give, and we must give back. This activity involves deciphering and meeting a pet's physical, psychological, and spiritual needs. Let's take a look at these requirements.

Physically, we have to feed our pet appropriately, even figuring out a special diet if necessary. My oldest son's dog has about a five-food palate. Other foods make her sick. And of course, pets require movement and exercise, depending on their species, as well as shelter.

Emotionally, most pets require bonding time. The amount depends on their species but also their personality. I know that cats are said to be aloof, but my cat Johnny, who lived with me a few years ago, insisted on sleeping on my chest every night. He absolutely loved being cuddled and would purr half the night. As another example, my son once had five goldfish. They followed his face around the tank whenever he peered in but drifted about aimlessly when he was gone. I'm certain they saw a special sort of light in my son. Love is always the best nourishment.

Just as pets share psychic information with us, they sometimes require the same. Upon arriving home from traveling—and this is years ago—I would find Max, my guinea pig, frenetic and frantic. This was quite unlike him. At all other times, Max was calm and collected.

He needed to be. Max ran the household. From his cage in the dining room, he could see everything happening on the top floor of the house. Frequently, the dogs and cat would stop at his cage, cock their heads, and set off in a new direction, Max having dictated marching orders. Even Wilma, my wandering turtle, as well as my friends' visiting pets, would pause at the cage and check in.

I decided to help Max out.

Before returning from one particular trip, I sent Max a psychic missive. Using the pet communication tools that you'll learn in chapter 5, I told him to get the house ready. When I walked through the door a day later, Max was cool and serene—and the dogs and cat were lined up in the dining room like well-behaved schoolchildren. I surmised that Max took his management job so seriously that he was upset when I arrived home and he hadn't had time to prepare the troops. From then on, I always gave Max due notice when coming home from a trip.

As I'll share in chapter 8, I believe that Max, although he has passed on, continues to manage the household. Now he's even more powerful, though. Once pets move beyond the body, their true nature can shine even stronger.

Pets can also relay their needs to us intuitively. A few years ago, one of my clients was struck with a panic attack. For the next hour, representations of fire appeared in her environment. A house on a television show burst into flames. Her son lit a match, which he wasn't supposed to do. She heard three fire truck sirens through the open window. Not knowing what was up, she meditated and perceived a psychic image of her horse, which she boarded at a nearby farm. Frantically, she called the boarding manager and asked if there was a problem at the farm.

"No," said the manager.

My client pushed until the manager agreed to check the horse stalls. The phone went dead, and he called back an hour later. Apparently, one of the groomers had dropped a burning cigarette near a haystack, starting a fire that could have quickly grown out of control. My client's horse had saved the day: it had sent the smell of smoke to my client, who had then interpreted the sign.

Sometimes it's hard to figure out if the origin of a psychic message is a pet or a human. I once worked with a client whose rabbit kept throwing up. The vomiting stopped as soon as my client discovered she was pregnant and her morning sickness set in. Mr. Rabbit had been mirroring his human companion's condition.

Is it really possible for our pets to relate to us psychically, if not spiritually? I believe that not only do pets have souls, but that they are conscious, or able to perceive and act with awareness. Recent research by neuroeconomics professor Gregory Burns shows that a key brain region, found in both humans and dogs, operates in a similar fashion. This is the caudate nucleus. Rich in dopamine receptors, this gland is known as a "consciousness center," regulating positive emotions like love and attachment. The fact that a dog's caudate nucleus functions at the same level as does that of a human child suggests that dogs are sentient (Dvorsky 2013).

Mammals and rodents also have a fully developed caudate nucleus. Birds have a somewhat similar brain circuitry and are also considered to perform at a high level of consciousness. Neurologically, reptiles and amphibians have a lesser-developed brain system and are believed to be less conscious, but still conscious. For instance, they exhibit a sort of primary consciousness (Butler and Cotterill 2006), a survival instinct that is sometimes intuitive in nature. As these studies suggest, the neurological wiring exhibited by humans and their pets might explain some of the reasons that we can be spiritually and even psychically connected.

As displayed, we must be ever-attuned to the two-way relationship between ourselves and our pets. The exchange of care can help us correct the disturbances that humans have caused the nonhuman nations over the ages, but it accomplishes much more than this. The pet/human bond is key to fulfilling our independent and mutual destinies. To understand the importance of this relationship, it's necessary to consider the path of the individual pet soul, the subject of the next section.

A Pet's Journey Across Time

Once upon a time, all beings dwelled together in heaven. No one hurt each other. Knowledge was granted before it was needed. Heaven was sublime because spirits occupied it. Your spirit—and that of your pet—is the immortal essence that knows itself as completely connected to the Spirit.

We use many names for the Spirit, including God, Christ, the Goddess, Allah, the One, Creator Consciousness, the Universe, Ganesh, Kwan Yin, and more. In this book, I'll most often use the phrase "the Spirit" and sometimes "the Creator." You can substitute a different name if you like. The names are varied, but our combined knowledge of this being or force is always of love, grace, and mercy. The spiritual aspect of ourselves and our pets still understands that it is bonded with the Spirit. Hence, our spirits can't help but perceive the world through the lens of love and act accordingly.

Paradise was wonderful, but it was also somewhat boring. The nature of the Creator is to create through generating more love. Made in the image of the Creator, all spirits shared these same yearnings. And so, each spirit journeyed forth into the expanding universe, which was only starting to take form. Each expressed a unique set of spiritual qualities, such as honor, healing, truth, loyalty, justice, or happiness. These qualities became the basis for a spirit's spiritual purpose and its own special way of formulating more love, or re-creating heaven, in the emerging cosmos. Thus each spirit reflected a dharmic purpose, its special calling or spiritual directive. We'll frequently speak about ways to support your pet's personal dharma in this book.

It wasn't enough to merely spread love. Spirits also wanted to experience it. To do so, a spirit needed to be able to choose between "love" and "not love." Innately, a spirit can't be anything but loving, so each spirit crafted a soul, a sort of slowed-down version of itself. A soul can act lovingly or not. The consequence of failing to come from love rather than fear and greed spelled disaster. Over time, souls became traumatized and they traumatized others, incurring and causing wounds and dysfunctional beliefs.

The entrance of darkness and suffering initiated several changes for souls. In order for a soul to achieve its dharmic purpose, which it was still charged to do, a soul also had to attend to its negative experiences and beliefs. In other words, it needed to work through its karma, which may be defined as the events and perceptions creating distorted views about love but also enabling loving knowledge and actions. Basically, souls had to start dealing with their karma in order to fulfill their dharma.

At about this point, souls started forming family or soul groups. In general, these were organized according to dharmic purpose. For instance, souls devoted to truth created one family; those dedicated to honesty, another family. In this way, souls could support each other in fulfilling their purpose. They could also assist each other with working through their often-similar karmic patterns. Most of these soul groups still exist today, although these groups have been further delineated. For instance, we'll now find a soul group consisting of the cat tribe, another composed of centipedes, and yet another for humans.

In order to catalog all their karmic experiences, misperceptions, and lessons, another change occurred. Each soul developed a mind. The mind is like a non-local computer that keeps track of everything the soul has learned or still has to learn. But even the activity of thinking things through wasn't enough to clear karma. To really gain knowledge about love, souls required hands-on learning, so they started incarnating in physical bodies, or lifetimes.

A lifetime serves as an organized lesson plan composed of specific karmic tasks and dharmic undertakings. I believe that most of the souls that are alive right now have already experienced previous lifetimes in different universes and also on this planet, reincarnation having become the standard protocol for managing karma and delivering dharma. At this point, I also believe that souls nearly always return in the same type of body, whether animal, vegetable, or human.

This doesn't mean that a tiger in one lifetime can't show up as a human or elephant in another. It can. I have a friend who remembers being a cornstalk. However, a soul is a set of frequencies or codes that combine to a unique self. Each nonhuman and human body is also composed of distinct codes. Over time, souls have tended to fixate in bodies that match their codes, which are based on karma, dharma, personality traits, and other factors. In fact, they also like to partner with the same souls; thus do many souls choose to meet up again, lifetime after lifetime. Once again, the causal reason is matching karma (personal history) and dharma (higher purpose).

You'll learn all about the codes that make up your pet's energetic signature, or unique personality, in chapter 2. For right now, the salient point is that you and your pet are connected for very important karmic and dharmic reasons. As a case in point, my dog Lucky is a reincarnation of my childhood dog named Muffy. How do I know? I had a dream in which Muffy appeared, barked, and then disappeared into the tubby body of Lucky the puppy. This occurred soon after we brought Lucky home.

I was glad that I was being given another chance to establish a healthy and loving bond with Muffy's soul because I'd always felt guilty about not taking good care of her when I was young. My mother had forced me to raise Muffy in the backyard. As I grew older, I seldom played with her. I'm now more than making up for the lack of attention I'd given Muffy back then through endless play dates with Lucky. As you can surmise, Muffy/Lucky and I are working through karma but also dharma. Lucky is teaching me about joy, and I am helping him learn how to trust. Actually, I wouldn't be surprised to discover that Muffy/Lucky had once been a member of one of my ancestor's families. I'll present an example of this phenomenon in chapter 8, when I more thoroughly explore my complicated relationship with Honey, my other dog.

There is another explanation for the reason that souls connect with us in one lifetime after another. When a soul is incarnating, whether as a natural or human being, its karmic and dharmic patterns are uploaded into its subtle and physical anatomies; you'll learn about these structures in the next section. Yet another type of energy can also be transferred into a body from the soul. It's called an attachment, and I'll thoroughly explore this structure in upcoming chapters. Right now, it's enough to know that attachments are subtle contracts that connect souls across time and space. Remaining in place beyond death, they operate like ropes that tie two or more souls together. Inevitably, these souls are pulled into each other's orbits and replay the same scenarios, lifetime after lifetime, until one or more party frees itself. Freedom essentially involves working through the karmic reasons the souls are intertwined.

For example, I have a client who was scared that he would hurt his cat, which was beloved by his wife, because it shrieked in the middle of the night. Fortunately, he came to see me before he did so. We figured out that the three of them—the man, wife, and cat's soul—had incarnated several times before. During each incarnation, the man had murdered the cat because he was jealous of the way his wife felt about it. The current incarnation of the cat screamed at night because it was afraid of getting killed again. As I expected, there was an attachment between all three souls. This binding disintegrated after my client dealt with his jealousy and decided to be more loving toward his wife *and* his cat—and the cat stopped freaking out at night.

How does the soul maintain these complicated storylines? In a nutshell, everything occurs because of energy: the good, bad, ugly, and beautiful. Because of this, it's important to understand the basic concepts and functions of energy, our next topic. Only by shifting energy can we help our pets—and ourselves—work through karma and trauma and realize our individual and common destinies. Only by operating energetically can we reengage and finally fulfill the covenant between the nonhuman and human nations.

It's a Matter of Energy
(And Energy Is What Matters)

Energy is information that moves, and everything occurs because of it. In fact, every time you touch, feed, or praise your pet, you are interacting with it energetically. Whenever you sense a pet's fear, tune in to its pain, or hear its "voice" in your head, you are engaging energetically. No matter what is happening with your pet, yourself, or between the two of you, it's a matter of energy. The trick to altering the negative energy causing bad situations—and to enabling uplifting energy toward creating great situations—is discerning between the two basic types of energy, which are physical and subtle.

Physical energy is measurable and concrete. We comprehend physical energy through our five senses, which are hearing, seeing, tasting, touching, and smelling. The fact that we can share our experiences of physical energy—i.e., if I'm seeing a cowboy hat, you will as well—makes it highly predictable. In regard to pets, this means that if you feed your pet, their hunger will be satiated. If you tell a dog to fetch, they ought to. (Unless they are my dogs, of course. They will simply raise their eyebrows. Even that reaction is predictable, I guess.)

Most books aim at improving a pet's life and a pet/human relationship by explaining how to analyze and shift physical energy. This book will do some of that as well. If your pet is exhibiting behavioral, psychological, or physical issues, you'll need to calculate, problem-solve, and monitor for change through physical means. You might have to take the pet to a vet, nurture them more lovingly, or train them better. The caveat is that most of the situations that appear in physical reality actually stem from events occurring in the subtle realms. You see, subtle energies dictate the activity of physical energies.

As compared to physical energies, subtle energies are less measurable and predictable. Hence, we can't perceive subtle energies on an X-ray machine or with the naked eye. Other words that mean subtle energy hint at its supernatural behavior, such as psychic, mystical, intuitive, and spiritual energy. Yet other terms equating with subtle energy include zero point, etheric, and quantum energy; and orgone, scalar waves, biophotons, tachyons, chi, prana, time-reversed waves, and biofields. The phrase "subtle energy" works for me because it was first used by Albert Einstein, who defined subtle energy as the "force remaining in the absence of all known forces" (Crowe 2004, 206).

What was Einstein getting at? He was suggesting that if you remove everything concrete from an object or situation, there is an energy underlying it. This is subtle energy, which formulates and sustains all of physical reality. This means that if you want to improve matters in concrete reality, from your pet's behavior to its health, you must alter what's happening in the related subtle reality.

I've found that pets are highly sensitive to what's occurring between the physical and subtle realms, and most of my friends and clients agree. For instance, I have a client whose iguana, Ralph, suddenly developed spots right before her son caught the measles. As soon as the child's spots appeared, the iguana's spots disappeared. It seemed as if Ralph was trying to warn the family that the child was getting sick. One of my dogs, Honey, spent four days lying in bed after my son had surgery for a deviated septum and polyps. Honey only rose to go outside when my son went to the bathroom. He was providing my son both physical and emotional support. Yet another time, I came home sad. I had just dropped my son off at college. To my surprise, Honey greeted me at the door with five squeaky toys. They were laid in a row. One at a time, he picked up each toy and squeaked it. Psychically sensing from afar that I was sad, he had planned a celebratory way to cheer me up.

While physical and subtle energies are interdependent, different bodies of science explain each type of energy. The classical laws of science, which describe the ways that objects interact with forces, police physical energy. In general, classical science says, "What you see is what you get." If you give a dog a bone, that bone soon will be reduced to rubble. If you give a kitty catnip, it will be amused for hours. Subtle energy, on the other hand, is described by quantum mechanics, which is the study of quanta, the smallest units of the universe. Quanta are labeled "freaky" or "spooky" because quantum laws aren't very rule-bound, at least not by classical standards.

In quantum reality, an object exists in at least two places at a time and only physically appears when—and where—it is observed. This means that subtle energy can be steered by the power of choice, or intentional focus. This suggests that when dealing with your pet, you can influence anything from your pet's behavior to its spiritual development by becoming conscious of what is happening on the subtle level. By subsequently shifting the subtle energies—or consciously visualizing a beneficial outcome—the physical energies will then respond.

Another quantum rule is that two objects, having met, remain entangled, or connected. This means that two objects or beings will continue influencing each other, even if separated by time and space. For example, if you are in a rotten mood, your pet might become grumpy. Then again, if you are unhappy, your pet might pick you up by becoming cheery. Because time and space don't interfere with connectivity, the law of entanglement also explains how your pet can contact you once it's deceased, as well as how you find each other, lifetime after lifetime. Once bonded, our souls remain linked.

Besides understanding the main differences between physical and subtle energies, it's also necessary to know about their differing anatomies. Physical energy is governed by the physical anatomy, which is composed of physical organs, channels, and fields. The organs include the liver and gallbladder, among others. The channels include the blood and lymph vessels. Physical fields emanate from every atom, cell, and organ. These fields are basically composed of electromagnetic and sonic frequencies, or light and sound.

In turn, subtle energies are run by the subtle anatomy, which is comparable to the physical anatomy in that it's also constituted by organs, channels, and fields. The subtle structures are similar to physical systems in that their job is to process energy. And what energies do they manage but light and sound? In comparison to the physical anatomy and their correlated energies, the light and sound governed by the subtle structures simply move faster or slower, obey quantum rather than classical laws; and are directed by consciousness rather than physical manipulation.

In terms of the subtle systems referenced in this book, we'll work the chakras, meridians, and auric fields. All three subtle systems organize subtle energy but can also convert subtle into physical energies and vice versa. This means that subtle systems are energetic transformers. You'll discover exactly how important this function is in this book when you're busily translating a pet's feelings into understandable thoughts or sending love to clear a microbial disease.

Mainly, however, we'll be focused on the chakras, the same subtle organs befriended by the long-ago Hopi and hundreds of other cultures. Each chakra manages a certain set of physical, psychological, and spiritual considerations, but they are hardwired from the get-go to reflect the unique temperament of a pet's soul. In fact, the soul front-loads each chakra with unique karmic and dharmic programs during and just before conception. As a lifetime ensues, chakras then incorporate additional programs and ideas, including derivatives of familial beliefs, personal experiences, and environmental factors. In short, we could say that a chakra is a sort of "mini brain," a storage house of memories and energies. Because of this, we can analyze and problem-solve for almost any concern through the chakras. We'll do a more formal "meet and greet" of the chakras in chapter 3. For now, understand that your pet's chakras are already at work, percolating with subtle energies that simply need a little attention to improve matters.

As stated, we'll also be interacting with two other well-known subtle structures in this book, the meridians and auric fields. Meridians are channels that carry an energy called *chi* in Traditional Chinese Medicine. Running through the connective tissue, the twelve main meridians distribute chi through the subtle and physical systems, delivering nourishment and clearing congestion. In chapter 7 we'll focus on one particular meridian. I want you to experience the ease and power of using meridian-based therapy on pets.

The auric field is composed of twelve auric fields, also called layers, which encircle the body. Each field is actually an extension of a chakra. Generated from the skin outward, these fields slightly overlap, each serving as a representative of its related chakra. In general, the fields are ordered in the same sequence as their chakra kin, except that the tenth auric field lies over the first auric field, which is located within and just outside of the skin. The second auric field follows, and so on. Finally, the ninth field is followed by the eleventh, with the twelfth auric field situated atop the eleventh. Based on the programming within a chakra, each layer determines which subtle energies will enter the body. Every layer also sends chakra-programmed subtle messages into the world, thus encouraging the world to respond in certain ways.

As stated, both physical and subtle structures process light and sound. In regard to chakras, each functions on a distinct band of light, which can be interpreted as a color. Every chakra also emanates specific sounds, which can be reduced to a tone. In this book you'll learn how to assess the relative health of a pet's chakra by comparing its coloration or tonality to its baseline. You'll also be shown how to send colors and tones into a pet's chakra so as to create balance and therefore more physical, psychological, and spiritual well-being. The great debate, when it comes to chakra colorations, is this: Exactly what colors describe the top in-body chakras?

Chakra	Color	Purpose
1	red	survival, security
2	orange	emotions, creativity
3	yellow	mentality, structure
4	green	relating, healing
5	blue	communicating, clairaudience
6	violet	vision, clairvoyance
7	white	spirituality, consciousness
8	black or silver	mysticism
9	gold	higher purpose, harmonizing
10	brown	grounding, earth connections
11	pink	supernatural and natural forces
12	clear	unique to each purpose

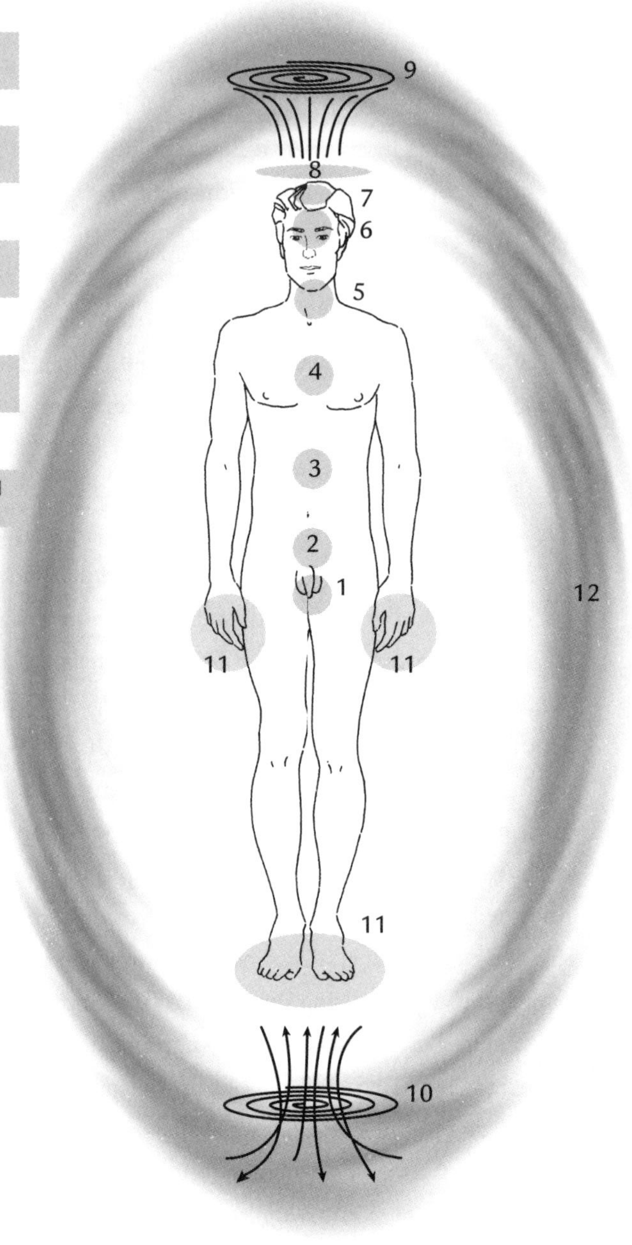

Figure 1: The Human Twelve-Chakra System

Both humans and pets have a twelve-chakra system.
This figure depicts the human chakra system.

From the coccyx upward, the colors assigned the lower five in-body chakras are red, orange, yellow, green, and blue. Some chakra experts believe that the sixth chakra, located in the brow, is indigo, and that the seventh chakra, at the top of the head, is violet. I perceive the sixth chakra as violet and the seventh chakra as white. My conclusion is based on research performed by Dr. Valerie Hunt back in the 1970s, which revealed that each of the seven in-body chakra functions within a band of colored lights that described the top two chakras as violet and white (Hunt et al, n.d.). If your opinion differs, simply convert my depiction of the chakra colors to your own.

Figure 1 depicts the twelve-chakra system as it is found in humans. You can use this illustration when focusing on your own chakras while interacting with a pet. Figures 2 and 3 show a mammal's chakra systems. You'll be able to compare the human and pet auric fields in chapter 3.

As you'll soon discover, interacting with the subtle energy system—your pet's and your own—will afford you unlimited ways to decipher and meet your pet's needs. You'll also be able to make positive shifts in your own well-being while improving the bond that already exists between you and your pet.

To be really prepared for the most interactive parts of this book, it's helpful to understand the spiritual attributes and qualities reflected by your pet. The matter of energetic codes and signatures is the subject of the next chapter. Turn the page to learn even more about our fellow kin, the nonhuman nations traveling this good green earth with us.

Chakra	Color	Purpose
1	red	survival, security
2	orange	emotions, creativity
3	yellow	mentality, structure
4	green	relating, healing
5	blue	communicating, clairaudience
6	violet	vision, clairvoyance
7	white	spirituality, consciousness
8	black or silver	mysticism
9	gold	higher purpose, harmonizing
10	brown	grounding, earth connections
11	pink	supernatural and natural forces
12	clear	unique to each purpose

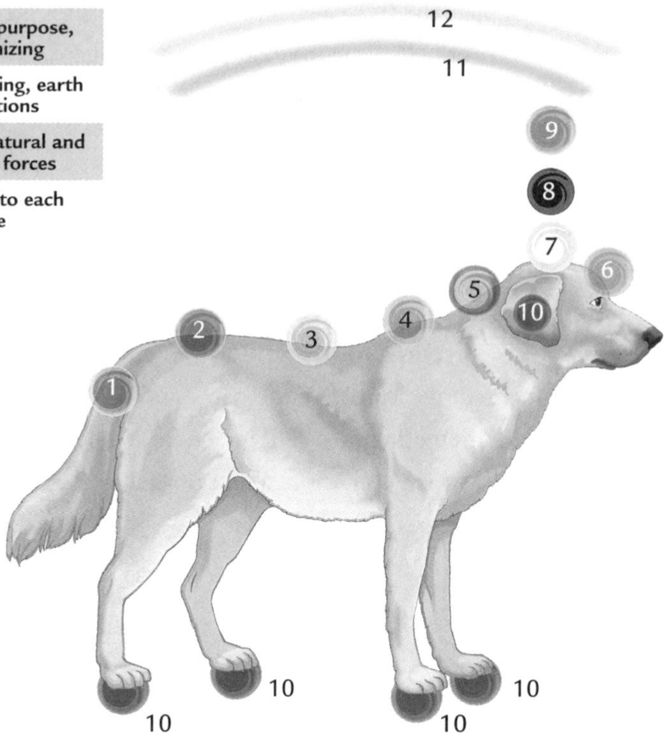

Figure 2: Mammal Chakras' Spinal and Out-of-Body Locations

The twelve chakras in all mammals, including rodents, are in the same bodily sites. This image showcases the locations of the seven in-body chakras in the spine and the five out-of-body chakras. The bud chakras are part of the tenth chakra. They are located under the ear area and under the feet. The bud chakras enable perception of environmental vibrations and noises.

Chakra	Color	Organ/Tissue
1	red	adrenals
2	orange	ovaries, testes
3	yellow	pancreas
4	green	heart
5	blue	thyroid
6	violet	pituitary
7	white	pineal
8	black or silver	thyroid (also linked to shoulder blades)
9	gold	diaphragm
10	brown	bone marrow, bud chakras
11	pink	muscles, connective tissue
12	clear	connected to 21 secondary chakras

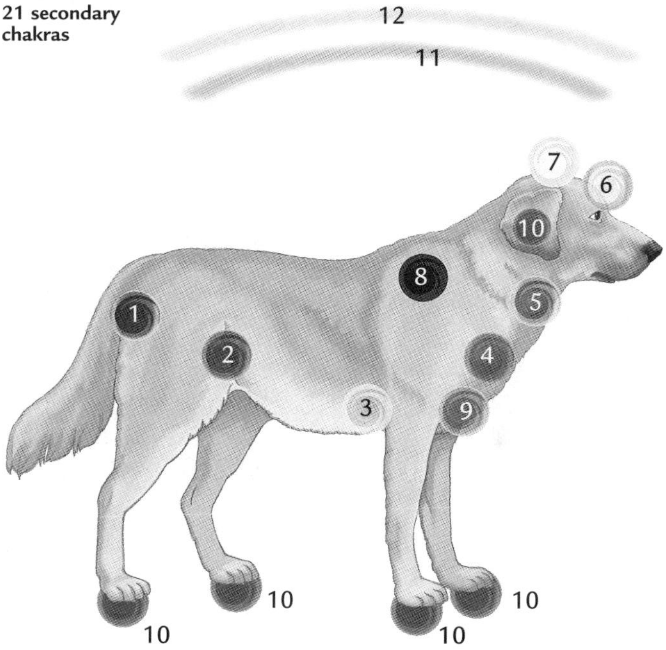

Figure 3: Mammal Chakras' In-Body Locations

This image shows the locations of the twelve chakras
in relation to their major organs.

Chapter Two
Your Pet's Personal Energetic Signature

Uniqueness is like a signature;
nobody can forge its exact copy.

Michael Bassey Johnson

The court of law allows identification based on a person's signature. There is a very different type of signature that explains the true nature of our pets; it's called an energetic signature. There are basically three different types of energy codes that add up to your pet's all-inclusive energetic signature. Understanding a pet's overall signature can key you in to its true nature, help you best decide what type of healing or support to offer, and encourage growth in both the pet and the self.

An energetic signature is a subtle energy code or imprint. Your pet's overarching signature is composed of three different sets of codes, which are carried by the soul and expressed through the body:

Categorical codes: This code is defined by a pet's membership in a pet category. The categories are mammals, rodents, birds, reptiles, arthropods, amphibians, and aquatic fish.

Species codes: Each of the seven categorical groups breaks into different species, which reflect specific character traits.

Personal codes: Every soul has undergone a distinctive set of experiences. These interactions have created a personal code, which is a complicated mix of karma, dharma, personality quirks, and life experiences.

Before discussing these matters, I'll first explore the spiritual basis for the existence of pet signatures. This conversation will highlight a few of the cultures that have ascribed traits to natural beings across time. Then, after showcasing each of the three types of codes affiliated with a pet's soul, I'll teach you a technique vital to all practices in this book. It's called Spirit-to-Spirit, and it's one of my signature techniques. Finally, you'll use Spirit-to-Spirit, as well as a pencil and paper, to compose your pet's overall energetic signature. You can conduct this exercise for every pet you currently interact with and also pets that have passed.

The Mystical Tradition Explaining Pet Signatures

There is a long-standing and ancient tradition that supports our view of pets as reflecting specific and special traits. In fact, hundreds of cultures across time have believed in "totemism," which portrays humans as enjoying a mystical kinship with a member of a nonhuman nation, such as an animal or a plant. By understanding totemism, you can better comprehend how your pet reflects general and specific characteristics that hold meaning for you.

A totem is a natural being, either in physical or spiritual form, or a sacred object or symbol that depicts a being. Other words for totem include tutelary spirit, power animal, power spirit, and spiritual guide, all referring to a being that serves either a group of people—such as an entire clan, tribe, or family—or a single person. Usually appearing in spirit form, the totem offers protection, guidance, and warnings. It can also represent the inner nature of a group or person, often reminding them that they carry the same qualities as the totem.

A group totem is frequently illustrated in a clan's legends or myths that depict an important event, such as a migration or a victory. Individuals within that group might showcase the totem as a tattoo, on clothing, or through art. This tradition is common in Africa, India, Oceania, and parts of North and Central America, as well as amongst the Australian Aboriginals (Haekel, n.d.).

I find the Australian Aboriginals' explanation of totemism one of the most interesting, as it is founded in the Aboriginal belief in Dreamtime. The Dreaming was a sacred era in which patterns were laid physically and subtly upon the earth. These patterns are blueprints for living in concert with nature. Each pattern is regulated by a totem that represents a set of beliefs. For instance, there are Shark, Honey Ant, and Kangaroo Dreamings. Each of these and the other totem Dreamings differ and can be explained by the characteristics and features of the natural being.

During the fifth month of a pregnancy, a soul "dreams" its way into one of the holy Dreamings and then follows the related blueprint while alive. Thus the person develops the attributes of the totem, even while operating as custodian for the land managed by the related energy (Crystalinks, n.d.).

As implied, the totem can serve as an emblem but also as a source of principles and beliefs that "charges" a piece of land or a group. The same type of relationship can occur between a totem and an individual. The main difference is that an individual's totem relationship is more intimate than that usually experienced by a group's members. Based on my own studies around the world, I have found that the totem/person relationship can be formed in many ways.

For instance, a family member or shaman can decipher a person's totem by paying close attention to events occurring around a child's birthing time. If a blue jay, tiger, hawk, or other natural being makes an obvious appearance, it can be considered a personal totem. Totemism always incorporates the understanding that every natural group reflects unique qualities, which I call codes, as do the specific beings that show up. Thus is the child's nature considered similar to the totem's nature; they might even be named after the totem. From this point on, if that being appears again, whether as a physical being or in a spiritual form, the person must pay particular attention to a situation and deal with it using the qualities reflected by the totem.

In many cultures, special events are organized to connect a person with a totem. The most well-known ritual is the vision quest. Most typically, a young person is left alone in the wilderness for three days and told to attend to their dreams, visions, and the visitations of natural beings. Whichever being makes the most pronounced appearance is considered a personal totem and will lend its assistance throughout the rest of that young person's life.

Many of my friends, clients, and students have engaged with personal totems. One of my friends connected with her totem while hiking in the mountains, where she came upon a bear. The bear stared at her, as if communicating, before ambling off. This friend now sees that particular bear in her dreams whenever she is in need of strength, one of the qualities represented by bears.

She swears it is the exact same bear, which means that she is bonded with that unique bear's soul.

Yet another client is affiliated with the snake. There isn't a specific snake that shows up in her everyday life or as an apparition. Rather, whenever she spies a snake in the real or dream world, she knows it's time to address a primal life concern, as that is one of the functions represented by snakes. You'll learn more about what snakes and other species symbolize in this chapter.

I have several totems. Most presented themselves through the mystical universe and continue to relate to me that way, but a certain type shows up in 3-D form, usually when I'm traveling and nervous because I'm in a precarious or unusual situation. For instance, I once journeyed alone across England to visit forty-four power sites. Most were located off the beaten track, such as in fields and caverns and along dirt roads. A storm suddenly arose when I was at the far end of a field. The wind was so strong that I had to huddle under a tree; I simply couldn't get back to the car. A dog with one blue eye and one brown eye showed up and comforted me, only leaving when the storm was over.

The same phenomenon occurred when a friend and I were trekking up a mountain in Belize. We were both feeling spooked, as if a wild animal were watching us. Again, a dog with two different eye colors appeared. It trotted alongside of us for about ten minutes and disappeared when we reached the top. This same type of dog—with two eye colors—has shown up about a dozen times in my adult life. As you'll learn in this chapter, dogs are loyal and protective. I believe that my need draws a particular type of dog—or totem—to me, no matter where I am. Why does my peculiar protector have two different colors of eyes? As you'll learn later in this chapter, in the section "Your Pet's Physical Characteristics," blue represents communication, and brown is earthy. My "security" dogs are basically communicating the fact that I am physically safe, and maybe they are even the reason that I am.

When a totem mirrors a part of our personality, it can point out traits that are already obvious or that lie dormant within us. But a totem can also exhibit complementary qualities, in which case that totem forms a powerful partnership with us. The most well-known example is the colloquial witch's cat.

Historically, a witch is usually a healer or similarly gifted person. Whether the witch's embodied assistant is a cat, dog, bird, bat, or other natural being, that being often supplements the witch's gifts. For instance, cats are sensitive to invisible spirits. A cat's reactions to the environment might clue the healer into a spiritual presence.

In this book we'll be working with pets, a special type of totem. A pet might serve as a sort of "familiar," which is the term used to describe a complementary partner, or stir a particular attribute within you. A pet might be alive or deceased, but no matter what, all members of a nonhuman nation that enter our lives carry energies that we need to be around and learn from.

Categorical Codes
Classifications of Conduct

In school we learned about different categories of natural beings, such as amphibians, mammals, and reptiles, among others. Technically, these groupings are called "classifications" or "classes," and it's a good thing that we have these summative genres, as there are up to one trillion species on this planet (Pappas 2016). It's far simpler to describe the characteristics of a group rather than the traits of thousands or millions of group members.

In this book I'm going to present categories that cluster the most common pets, which are mammals, rodents, birds, reptiles, arthropods, amphibians, and aquatic fish. The reason that I'm writing an entire section about the aptitudes of these seven classifications is that pet souls reflect the features or signatures of their principal group. In fact, I believe that many pet souls enter a specific type of natural body because they desire to experience and express the qualities exhibited within that class.

There are many reasons why a pet's soul is attracted to a certain classification. They might already be comfortable with the related attributes. They might need to stimulate the related traits, as these features are latent within their soul. Then again, they might not have the slightest clue about these qualities but know that they must acquire them. In other words, your pet may or may not be "good at" the codes attributed to their classification.

For instance, in this chapter you'll learn that birds represent freedom. This could lead you to wonder why your pet bird huddles in its cage, too scared to fly. Don't be impatient. Your pet might not have had previous experiences with freedom. It takes a long time to become adept, or even okay, at something new.

Know too that classifications have built-in features but also front-loaded limitations. Limitations are the cost of learning about love. Limitations aren't all bad. When we are limited, we are forced to make decisions that are wise. As you'll discover in this section, mice are great at details, but they are way too tiny to see the big picture. You can't expect a pet mouse to grasp what's happening in the entire household, only to notice what's in front of them.

The next section is a rendering of the seven pet categories we're covering in this book. In it, I'll describe the codes most prevalent in each category and provide keywords to help you remember the designated codes. I'll also offer a statement recognizing the main teaching being learned and taught by the beings in these categories. Then, because I recognize that you are probably working on some of the attributes featured by your pet, I'll present a question to help you evaluate your progress.

Near the end of this chapter, we'll loop back to this data and work with the information.

Mammals

Mammals, such as dogs and cats, are tribal in nature. They are clannish and quite affectionate and caring towards others, including humans. They are also protective and loyal, recognizing the needs of others. Mammals carry deep wisdom and are highly trustworthy.

> **Keywords:** tribal, loving
>
> **Main Teaching:** How to be warm and loving. Ask yourself if you err toward being too loyal or the opposite, which is cold and detached.

Rodents

Rodents, including mice and hamsters, are devoted to detail and the simplicity of the moment, paying attention to what is right in front of them.

> **Keywords:** detail, focus
>
> **Main Teaching:** Rodents ask us to live in the present moment, paying attention to details without getting overwhelmed. Ask yourself if you get lost in details or overlook them.

Birds

Birds illustrate freedom from earthly anchors and the transcendence of the soul. They ask us to choose a direction that is divinely approved.

> Keywords: freedom, transcendence
>
> Main Teaching: Birds prompt us to align our free will with the Spirit's will. Ask yourself if you are overindulging in freedom of choice or are hampered by fears and restrictions.

Reptiles

Reptiles are amongst the oldest living forms of life on this planet. They also reflect our reptilian brain, the ancient part of our neurology that governs survivalist responses. They invite us to embrace the desire—and right—to survive but also to make decisions based on ancient wisdom. As well, they reflect the most primal cycles of life, such as birth, death, and rebirth.

> Keywords: survival, transformation
>
> Main Teaching: Reptiles, including snakes, live according to primal rules, yet they are able to transform. Ask yourself if you are overly insecure or too ambitious.

Arthropods

Arthropods, like spiders and crabs, are invertebrates, which means they lack backbones. They symbolize pliability when divining one's personal destiny and the ability to create a path forward. Arthropods also shift between various physical and spiritual realms and are connected to the Faery realm.

> Keywords: destiny, dream-shifting (the ability to move between realms)
>
> Main Teaching: Arthropods focus us on our destiny, enabling a shift in perception so we can fulfill our goals. Ask yourself if you are accessing the intuitive knowledge required to fulfill your destiny or if you are "tuned out."

Amphibians

Amphibians, including frogs and newts, dwell in water and on land and merge the qualities of both. Water represents feelings, cleansing, flow, and intuition, and earth symbolizes groundedness, logic, and dependability. One of life's greatest mysteries is how to marry these seemingly different attributes.

> Keywords: flow, groundedness

> Main Teaching: Amphibians attune us to our emotions and intuitive guidance even while encouraging practicality. Ask yourself if you are overly emotional and psychic or too rational and practical.

Aquatic Fish

Across a variety of cultures, fish have represented inspiration, prophecy, and evolution. They also serve the sacred feminine and grant good luck.

> Keywords: inspiration, luck

> Main Teachings: Fish energy requests that we open to the divine feminine and her nourishment. Ask yourself if you are connected to the feminine aspects of the Spirit, inviting maternal- and self-nourishment, or if you are disconnected from your needs.

Species Codes

All the Many Offerings

As known by cultures invested in totemism, every species reflects noteworthy qualities or energetic codes. These properties are fairly obvious, based on a species' lifestyle. For instance, parrots love the sun, which makes them harbingers of illumination. They mimic humans, which makes them a sort of ambassador.

What special attributes or signatures are innate to your pet's species? What limitations accompany the positive traits? To analyze both, I invite you to study the chart in this section. You'll apply this information to your particular pet and yourself at the end of this chapter.

CHART: *Signatures and Limitations of Specific Pet Species*

Category	Species	Positive Signatures (Traits include...)	Limitations (Species can be...)
Mammals	Dogs	Loyalty, reliability, friendliness, protectiveness, playfulness	Overly enduring of abuse
	Cats	Independence, wholeness, self-awareness, patience, psychism	Selfish, oversensitive
	Horses	Nobility, sensuality, stamina, goal orientation, ability to traverse lands of light and dark	Gun-shy, untrusting, oversensitive
	Rabbits	Fertility, sensitivity, awareness of dangers, ability to travel to underworld, knowledge of when to freeze, fight, or flee	Over-alert, easily scared
	Ferrets	Opportunism, cunning, ability to see what's hidden	Revengeful, sneaky
	Pigs	Luck, intelligence, prosperity consciousness	Self-righteous, excessive
Rodents	Gerbils	Hardiness, sociability, appreciativeness	Clannish, attacking
	Hamsters	Fun-loving, responsible, ability to create opportunities	Overly worried, gluttonous
	Chinchillas	Innocence, warmth, ability to be silent	Overly "go with flow"
	Fancy rats	Ambitious, shrewd, creative	Gluttonous, lazy
	Guinea pigs	Intelligence, talkativeness, affectionate, ability to act as diagnostician and seer	Easily victimized
	Mice	Perfectionism, ability to focus, attend to details, and appreciate the small things in life	Fussy, overly analytical
Birds	Parakeets	Freedom; ability to mimic, create bonds, and act as messenger of gods	Copy-cattish; overly concerned with appearance
	Parrots	Uniqueness, joyfulness; ability to serve as emissary, truth teller, and harbinger of truth	Lacking in filters, bossy

Category	Species	Positive Signatures (Traits include...)	Limitations (Species can be...)
	Canaries	Sweetness, freshness; ability to perform healing and bring in fresh ideas and light	Too delicate, overly sensitive
	Macaws	Balancing, sociability; ability to understand others	Gossipy, too screechy
	Chickens	Boldness, enthusiasm, sociability, resourcefulness	Territorial, undiscerning
	Turkeys	Ability to honor nature, be abundant, and represent divine vision on earth	Adversarial, undiscerning
	Doves	Maternalism, nourishing, spiritual	Self-sacrificing
	Pigeons	Ability to deliver messages from angels and bestow divine blessings	Easily scapegoated
	Ducks	Diligence, contemplativeness; ability to be prepared yet go with flow	Overly vulnerable
	Geese	Bravery, loyalty, teamwork, fellowship; drive to protect the innocent	Silly, lazy, mean
Reptiles	Snakes	Ability to transform, serve ancient wisdom, perform healing, represent primal energy, and remain hidden unless provoked or endangered	Survivalist, covert, violent
	Lizards	Mystical and regenerative powers; adaptability and agility; ability to change colors or otherwise respond when endangered	Stealthy, secretive
	Iguanas	Stoicism, ease of motion, intuitiveness, contentment; ability to provide insight and camouflage	Secretive
	Turtles	Wisdom, emotional fluidity, persistence, peacefulness	Overly resistant or vulnerable

Category	Species	Positive Signatures (Traits include...)	Limitations (Species can be...)
Arthropods	Spiders	Ability to perceive destiny, create structure, and weave light with dark	Stealthy, dangerous
	Tarantulas	Ability to perceive destiny, create structure, keep perfect timing, and set up intelligent ambushes	Overly dominant
	Crabs	Self-protectiveness; being ambulatory; abilities to be maternal, flow cyclically, and represent weakness that must be protected	Overly guarded, reticent
	Ants	Hard-working, strength, responsible; ability to bring dreams into reality	Lacking in self-focus
	Caterpillars	Quickness; ability to transform and achieve hidden potential	Easily stuck, unable to change
	Centipedes	Coordination, busyness	Awkward
Amphibians	Frogs	Spiritual cleansing, prosperity; ability to perform alchemy and attract true love	Overly vulnerable or emotional
	Newts	Same as salamander, plus ability to perform witchcraft	Manipulative
	Salamanders	Magicality; ability to transform and reveal secrets	Overly solitary or secretive
	Toads	Sorcery ability; protectiveness (can use poison); operate through androgyny	Pompous under stress, overly servile
Aquatic	Fish, saltwater	Ability to swim in currents of life, achieve emotional and spiritual balance, and surround others in the healing power of the Divine Mother's womb	Overly emotional, lacking in masculinity
	Fish, freshwater	Ability to enjoy and flow with the currents of life, achieve emotional and spiritual balance, and apply clarity and purity toward healing purposes	Overly emotional, lacking in spiritual clarity

Category	Species	Positive Signatures (Traits include...)	Limitations (Species can be...)
	Angelfish	Beauty; ability to connect to spiritual guides and use color for healing	Jealous, self-aggrandizing
	Goldfish	Harmonizing, beauty; ability to create opportunities	Selfish, greedy
	Rainbow fish	Hopefulness, tolerance, equality; ability to deliver rewards after hardship	Lacking in self-definition
	Koi	Perceptivity; prosperity consciousness; delivery of ancient wisdom	Prideful, unfocused
	Guppies	Joyfulness; ability to transmit cultural wisdom	Foolhardy
	Seahorses	Gracefulness, masculine love, chivalry	Overprotective
	Sea snails	Ease, slowness, cleansing	Sluggish
	Betta fish (Siamese fighting fish)	Protection, boundaries, confrontation of ego, warriorism	Over-aggression, violence

How might you work with the above information as stand-alone data? I'll respond to this question by exploring betta fish, which are commonly called Siamese fighting fish.

Imported into the Western world from Thailand since 1910, bettas have become a very popular aquarium fish. They are beautifully colored, with long, flowing fins, and, though attractive, can be very aggressive. The males frequently fight each other, also attacking females after breeding. As for the females, if they are in too close a proximity with each other, they too might become hostile. The brutality is lessened in the wild when bettas have more space for swimming and can hide in solitude. Cramped quarters is one factor that leads to combat.

In fact, it is the aggressive nature of the bettas that brought them to the attention of the king of Thailand in the 1800s. Citizens were collecting and breeding bettas for fighting matches. The king became so interested in the competition that he sanctioned betta fighting events. Even now, some people breed the bettas, who are omnivores in nature, to battle each other.

Of course, most betta owners don't force their fish to fight—deliberately. But they do make other mistakes that can promote violence. Bettas attack if they don't have enough space. In most stores, you'll see them shoved into tiny little cups. Once taking them home, owners often fail to use large enough tanks or establish the proper separation between the bettas. Owners may believe that because bettas can eat plants, housing them with greens will sustain them; however, bettas need meat and protein to be healthy.

I share this background about the betta fish for three main reasons. First, the data I've provided serves as a sampling for the deep-dive research you should do when analyzing your pet's essential traits. All components of a pet's needs, attributes, and behavior add up to their species' code. Second, the richer the data, the more fodder you have to work with when figuring out what personality and soul traits you have in common with your pet. You'll perform both activities at the end of this chapter. Third, the gathered knowledge can advise you in how to treat—and not treat—your pet.

If you refer back to the previous chart, "Signatures and Limitations of Specific Pet Species," you'll see that I have summarized the data just shared. Betta fish can be aggressive, violent, and warrior-like. With the right boundaries and enough solitude, these battling traits can be nullified or controlled. If you are naturally attracted to betta fish, you most likely tend toward a certain amount of aggression and egoism, which you too can manage with appropriate boundaries and down time.

How do you accomplish these goals? Well, the same way that you support your betta fish. Pay special attention to your need for space and eat a well-balanced diet. Come up with ways to direct your warrior-like abilities toward positive ends and manage your reactions when people put *you* in a "tiny little cup" or a tight set of circumstances. You can learn all this and more because of your relationship with your betta fish—or whichever pet you are bonded with.

Now that you've become acquainted with the codes of the most popular pet species, it's time to delve into the particular and peculiar signatures of your pet.

Your Pet's Personal Codes

Anyone who has engaged with individuals from the same species can testify that they are not completely alike. I've had three turtles, and not one exhibited the same personality. Hercules was calm. Wilma was Amazonian. Willie was diminutive. I've also owned two white rats, Sleepy and Snoopy. They were named appropriately. Sleepy always snoozed. Snoopy played Red Baron. Literally, he would hang off the top of his cage and flap his paws, as if flying.

As implied by these examples, every pet has its own personal code (which is distinct from its energetic signature, which is cumulative). Carried on the soul but affected by events in the current life, this code is determined by the following factors:

- history, including past lives and in-between lives; history composes karma
- purpose, which is spiritual and creates dharma
- this-life experiences, involving several life stages
- a pet's personality quirks, which are unique to them
- physical characteristics, as affected by genes and the environment; these can shape physicality but also behavior and perception

Next, I'll explore each of these five basic areas in a jam-packed fashion. You'll work with this data in the last section of this chapter.

Your Pet's Karma

As already defined, karma reflects the sum total of a soul's experiences and mainly the lessons it must still learn to comprehend love. The soul loads karma into the pet's body just before and during conception. These ideas are altered and updated as a pet's life goes on.

No matter what a pet's karmic issues are, there are only two beliefs that the pet's soul and mind can hold about love. These are:

- I am separate.
- I am connected.

If a pet's soul believes itself separated from the Spirit, other spirits, and even its own spirit, it will exhibit behavioral, psychological, physical, and psychic signs of distress. It might act out or be overly shy; be emotionally shut down or reactive; or become ill, sick, or weak. It might also take on others' energies or create supernatural phenomena. The point of all exhibitions of separateness is to work them through. For example, I worked with a client whose cat was killed by a coyote when she was young. In fact, the cat died because my client had forgotten to bring it in one night. Consequently, she decided she wasn't trustworthy enough to ever own another animal. This is an example of a separating belief, as it is tainted with a lack of self-love.

One day, when my client was an adult, a stray cat pranced right through her front door, forcing her to adopt it. One night the cat snuck outside. Around midnight my client heard the cat screaming on the front lawn. She quickly ran to the door and the cat ran in the house, barely escaping a rampaging coyote. The cat doesn't wander anymore, having learned a karmic lesson, and my client isn't blaming herself for the cat's previous wanderings. In fact, both are starting to trust themselves and their bond. On nearly every level, the instant replay was karmic and based in separating beliefs. The end result, however, created connection.

Of course, not every challenging event is karmic. The physical body is prone to trials and illnesses. A pet can become ill, disturbed, or upset "just because." A pet's soul can also believe itself separate in one life area and not another. In general, however, a chronic or acute issue usually indicates a karmic lesson. Fundamentally, our pet's soul will do whatever it takes to know itself as connected to sources of love.

Your Pet's Dharma

What is your pet's essential purpose? What is your pet uniquely here to teach and reveal? While every single spirit, and therefore soul, is on earth to express a special form of love, there are fundamental categories of dharmic or spiritual giftedness. Most pets are on this planet to fulfill one or two of these purposes. As a clue, each of these purposes relates to a chakra, as you'll notice in chapter 3. Specifically, the dharmic purposes are linked with chakras one through eleven. This is because souls tend to live through one chakra more than others. The following list is written in the same order as the chakras and their stages, which are described in the next section. The twelfth chakra gift is unique to each pet, and its gifts are indescribable.

List of Pets' Dharmic Purposes

> Physical Dharma: Pet is very primal, physical, and active.
>
> Emotional Dharma: Pet meets the emotional needs of self and others.
>
> Mental Dharma: Pet is keenly intelligent and responsive to ideas.
>
> Relational Dharma: Pet is all about relationship and love, often serving as a healer.
>
> Communicative Dharma: Pet is communicative, expressive, and heeds verbal communiqués.
>
> Visual Dharma: Pet is devoted to the visual aspect of life and is usually clairvoyant.
>
> Spiritual Dharma: Pet is spiritually attuned and serves as a channel for spiritual truths.
>
> Mystical Dharma: Pet is a mini shaman. It is psychic and senses the presence of spirits and negative and positive energies.
>
> Harmonic Dharma: Pet helps everyone get along.
>
> Environmental Dharma: Pet is extremely aware of and sensitive to the environment, other natural beings, and natural events.
>
> Commanding Dharma: It seems that the pet runs everything and everyone around it.

As for how these dharmic patterns might appear in a pet, remember my former guinea pig, Max? Max definitely displayed command dharma. Everyone in the house responded to his cackling and nose pointing. My dog Honey is totally a communicator. If he's not barking, he's playing with a squeaky toy. When I travel, he still manages to wake me early in the morning with a psychic bark.

Think about what duties your own pet might be performing!

Your Pet's This-Life Experiences

As explained, your pet's soul carries previously obtained karma and dharma into every life. However, a new life brings new experiences, positive and negative. In order to continue developing, clear old karma, and express its dharmic purpose, a pet moves through several life stages. These are sequential and relate to developmental phases, such as conception or mid-maturity. In chapter 3 you'll discover that each stage also synchronizes to the active period of a particular chakra. We'll revisit the stages of development at several points in this book, as this knowledge can help you narrow down the inception of a trauma, better diagnose a pet's challenge, and even aid you in releasing your pet at death.

A Pet's Stages of Development

Stage One: Dharmic Selection. During preconception the spirit of the pet interacts with the Spirit to select the bodily programming and dharmic opportunities needed for the upcoming life.

Stage Two: Karmic Selection. During preconception the soul of the pet works with spiritual guides to help select the bodily programming and karmic lessons required for the upcoming life.

Stage Three: Programming. During conception the soul and spirit independently upload the selected karmic and dharmic information, respectively, into the subtle energy body. Both programs affect the genes and also the epigenetics, the chemical soup that surrounds the genes and holds ancestral memories. These programs will primarily affect the pet's relationship with the environment and surroundings.

Stage Four: Survival. During in utero through birth, parental issues and experiences are transferred into the pet's in utero body. Programs are chosen that will enhance physical survival.

Stage Five: Socialization. When an infant, the pet attunes to those around it, forming social skills.

Stage Six: Learning. When slightly older, the pet starts to put ideas together while testing its personal power within its environment and clan.

Stage Seven: Relating. When juvenile, the pet seeks and finds relationships mirroring its karma and dharma.

Stage Eight: Communicating. During early maturity the pet expresses its own needs and desires and pays attention to those verbalized by others.

Stage Nine: Self-Awareness. During middle maturity the pet starts making decisions based on personal preferences, although it might also mirror a human companion's issues. The observant companion can use this knowledge to improve themselves.

Stage Ten: Spiritualization. During late maturity a pet's most severe issues usually smooth out, leaving the pet more empathic and compassionate.

Stage Eleven: Supernatural Power. In early to mid-decline, being less ambulatory, the pet can (subconsciously) choose to access its supernatural abilities to relate to and help others. It might display mystical abilities or make things happen in unusual ways, such as through psychic visitations or by moving objects without touching them.

Stage Twelve: Transformation. During decline, dying, and into the afterlife, the pet's true nature is revealed as they prepare to die and then leave their bodies, and possibly communicate after death. During this stage a pet's soul is encouraged by the Spirit and its guides to claim and process their karmic and dharmic accomplishments.

One question I'm frequently asked is how these stages apply to a short-lived pet, such as a centipede, or what happens if the pet dies suddenly or when young. I'll talk about these issues more completely in chapter 8. Suffice it to say that every pet, no matter how long- or short-lived, can pass through every stage if it lives a full life. And if the death is unexpected, a pet's soul can fly through multiple stages in a split second. After all, the soul is made of subtle energy. In the quantum universe, infinite activities can occur in a moment.

However, a soul can also "freeze" at any stage. It might then fail to progress through that or later stages. This is common and usually occurs because of trauma. That's one of the reasons why you'll learn how to help heal a pet's trauma in several chapters of this book.

Your Pet's This-Life Personality Traits

Of course, your pet displays attributes that aren't explained by a formula. That's what makes them so interesting!

There are millions of descriptors, but they can be reduced to a few opposing active and passive traits. As you read through the examples, pay attention to your pet's characteristics. You'll work with this list at the end of the chapter.

CHART: *A Pet's Personality Traits*

Active Traits	Passive Traits
Busy	Lethargic
Skittish	Calm
Extroverted	Introverted
Risk-taker	Risk-averse
Open emotionally	Closed emotionally
Disagreeable	Agreeable
Expressive	Internal
Neurotic	Stable
Careless	Conscientious
Adventurous	Predictable
Affectionate	Separate
Humorous	Dry
Social	Independent

Not only do a pet's peculiarities define their personality, but their traits might also mirror your own. Studies show that people frequently share commonalities with their pets. For instance, owners of reptiles, which are highly independent, tend to be less social. Birds' human companions are usually as expressive as their birds, and cat lovers act much like their pet cats. Both are smart, introverted, nonconformist, and sensitive. Dog people, on the other hand, are frequently like dogs—extroverted, agreeable, conscientious, and lively. This might be because they need to walk their dogs and take them out and about, whereas bird and cat people don't need to do the same. And just like their fish, fish owners are happy people (Hubbard 2015). Of course, everyone is different. You can certainly love dogs and be an introvert. This interesting study does suggest, however, that your pet really might reflect your karma and dharma.

Your Pet's Physical Characteristics

When embodied, your pet's soul reflects the characteristics of its physical appearance as well as the environment. For instance, as a child I owned a green and blue parakeet that chatted nonstop. Anyone around that bird felt happier after meeting it. As you'll see, green is a healing trait, and blue connotes communication. The bird's coloration was sure on point! The following renderings of colors, marks, eyes, and stature/environmental conditions might help you better perceive how your pet reflects its particular characteristics.

CHART: *A Pet's Physical Characteristics and Their Meanings*

	Descriptor	Meaning
Colors	Red	Bold
	Orange	Creative
	Yellow	Mental
	Green	Relational
	Blue	Communicative
	Indigo	Integrity
	Purple	Imagination
	White	Purity
	Black	Mysticism
	Silver	Universally connected
	Gray	Private
	Gold	Powerful
	Brown	Earthy
	Taupe	Dependable
	Rose	Loving
	Neutral	Changeable
	Multi-colored	Dynamic
Marks	Brindle (tiger striped)	Ancestrally imprinted
	Striped (regular stripes)	Adaptable
	Spotted	Psychically protected
	Patchy	Fun-loving
	Dappled	Connected to heavens
	Marbled	Artistic yet stable
	Shimmery	Angelic
	Saddle or harness-like	Friend of the fairies
	Smooth	Serene

	Descriptor	Meaning
	Rough	Tough
Eyes	Blue	Calm, peaceful, knowledgeable
	Brown	Independent, self-aware
	Green	Curious, creative
	Hazel	Spontaneous, bold
	Black	Mysterious, shamanic
	Gray	Wise, gentle
	To interpret other eye colors, such as the yellows, reds, blues, and metallic silvers and golds found in birds or the blues, silvers, and blacks in goldfish, see the list of colors on page 50.	
Stature/ Environment		
	Low to ground	Earthy, practical
	High off ground	Perceptive
	Land-based	Sensible, functional
	Airborne	Heavenly, transcendent
	Water-based	Emotional, intuitive
	Tree- or plant-connected	Cheery, interconnected
	Likes heat	Fire energy is passionate and magical; the pet relies on an external source of life energy
	Likes cold	Produces own life energy

Certain species operate in more than one environment. For instance, a parakeet is connected to trees, although a pet parakeet uses a "perch-tree." It also flies in the air. Look up the meanings of "tree" and "air," and you'll discover that a parakeet serves up "heavenly cheer." You can put together similar configurations for your own pet.

How do you figure out if a pet is lower or higher to the ground? Perform a comparative analysis within its species. A dachshund is lower to the ground than a Dalmatian; therefore, it's more concerned with the everyday than would be its longer-legged friend.

Now that you are acquainted with some of the special characteristics of your pet, it's time to learn the technique that will help you form an energetic signature statement about your pet.

Exercise

Spirit-to-Spirit: Your All-Inclusive Technique

Spirit-to-Spirit is a one-size-fits-all technique for engaging intuitively. You'll be using it throughout this book for a variety of purposes, including assessing your pet's subtle energies, arriving at solutions to problems, and improving your pet/human bond. After introducing you to Spirit-to-Spirit, I'll immediately let you practice it. You'll employ this process to create the composite energetic signature of your pet.

Spirit-to-Spirit is conducted in three steps that invite only the highest level of information, provide energetic protection, and enable you to send and receive information and healing. The three steps and what they offer are as follows:

> **1: Affirm your personal spirit.** As already discussed, your spirit is your highest self. By acknowledging this aspect of you, you're requesting that only your best self is involved in any undertaking. To quickly conduct this step, it can be useful to imagine a picture or symbol that depicts your essential self, such as an angel, star, light, flame, or flower.
>
> **2: Affirm others' spirits.** Through this step, you're deciding to interact with the most essential aspect of someone or something else, including people, pets, animals, otherworldly beings, or any other entity or force. As with the previous step, you can formulate an image, envisioning others as angels, forms clothed in white, or beings that are smiling.
>
> **3: Affirm the Spirit.** Through this step, you are surrendering yourself and an activity to the Spirit. This requests that the Spirit will accomplish the following:
>
> - Formulate insights that are pure and correct.
> - Send messages when and how they are needed.
> - Guarantee accurate interpretations of intuitive and physical events and information.
> - Keep the others involved in a process safe and healthy.

- Protect you and others from inappropriate or harmful
  forces; also help you perceive intrusive forces so
  you can free yourself or another from them.

- Send healing and information to others, including a pet.

To acknowledge the Spirit, you can envision a picture, as you did in previous steps. Common examples include a white flame, a dove, the sun, the Christ, Mary, Ganesh, the Buddha, and other iconographic images.

Now you're ready to practice what was just preached.

Exercise
Creating Your Pet's Personal Energetic Signature

What is your pet's overarching energetic signature, and what might that signature suggest about your own vital nature or issues? In this exercise you'll use Spirit-to-Spirit to formulate a signature statement based on a pet's categorical, species-based, and personal codes. You'll be assessing yourself simultaneously so you can clearly understand how you are alike and unlike your pet. You'll summarize your findings in statements, one about your pet and one about you. In particular, the statement about your pet's energetic signature will help you assess and problem-solve for your pet. The statement about you will help you work on yourself and improve matters with your pet. You can use this exercise for every single pet you interact with, whether it is currently alive or not.

> *1: Prepare.* Gather paper and a writing instrument and make sure you
> won't be disturbed for about one hour. Select a quiet environment.

> *2: Conduct Spirit-to-Spirit.* Affirm your personal spirit, your pet's
> spirit, all helping spirits, whether visible or invisible, and the Spirit.
> Give permission for the Spirit to be your main source of insight and
> knowledge.

> *3: Assess the Categorical Code.* Return to page 35's section on
> categorical codes and focus on your pet's category: mammal,
> rodent, bird, reptile, arthropod, amphibian, or aquatic fish. Review
> the qualities ascribed to your pet. Label your paper "categorical
> codes." Then ask the Spirit to help you select and write down words
> or descriptors under that label in response to these three questions:

- What are the key categorical characteristics of my pet?

- How am I alike or unlike these traits?

- Am I too extreme in relation to any of
  these traits? In what ways?

Spend a moment reflecting on what you've discovered, then move on.

4: *Analyze for Species-Based Codes.* Return to page 38's section on species codes. Label your paper "species codes." Examine your pet's species, selecting any applicable positive characteristics and limitations. Request that the Spirit help you respond to the following queries:

- Which of the positive characteristics describe
  my pet? Are there additional ones to add?

- In what ways do any of the traits portray me?

- Which of the limitations describe my pet?

- Do any of these limitations depict me?

Consider what you've just learned about your pet and yourself, then move ahead.

5: *Create Your Pet's Personal Profile.* Re-examine page 44's section "Your Pet's Personal Codes." Label a section of your paper "personal codes," then respond to the questions related to each of the four previously outlined subsections.

- *Your Pet's Karma.* Questions are:

  Which of these two beliefs (separate / connected) does your pet seem to adhere to, and in what ways?

  Which of these two beliefs (separate / connected) do you abide by? Note related observations and thoughts.

  In what ways are you and your pet similar or dissimilar in regard to believing yourself separate or connected?

- *Your Pet's Dharma.* Review the eleven major
dharmic purposes, which are physical, emotional,
mental, relational, communicative, visual,
spiritual, mystical, harmonic, environmental, and
commanding. Now respond to these questions:

    Which of the dharmic purposes best matches my pet?

    Which of them best suits me?

    How is my pet's purpose and my own
    purpose similar or dissimilar?

- *Your Pet's This-Life Experiences.* Read through "Your Pet's This-Life
Experiences" beginning on page 46 and put a commiserate label
on your paper. Review the twelve stages of a pet's life and figure
out which one your pet is in, then respond to these questions:

    How has my pet moved through all
    stages before the current one?

    How is my pet dealing with the current stage?

    Is my pet stuck anywhere?

    How does my progress through life
    relate to my pet's development?

- *Your Pet's This-Life Personality.* Review page 49's section
"Your Pet's This-Life Personality Traits" and label
a section of your paper "personality traits." Now
review the active and passive personality traits and
write down your responses to these questions:

    Which active or passive traits depict my pet?

    Are there additional traits that apply to my pet?

    Which active or passive traits describe me?

    How am I alike or not alike my pet?

- *Your Pet's Physical Characteristics.* Refer back to page 50 and respond to the following questions.

  Colors: What color/s are my pet, and what does this mean?

  Marks: Which marks does my pet have, if any, and what do these marks indicate?

  Eyes: What color are my pet's eyes, and what does that say about my pet?

  Stature/environment: What does my pet's stature or the listed environmental factors reveal about my pet?

  Self: How do my pet's traits relate to me? (You can also self-reflect on colors, as per your hair and eyes, in relation to yourself.)

6: ***Compose Your Pet's Personal Energetic Signature.*** Review what you've written; now you'll be putting everything together. In regard to your pet, compose a simple statement or paragraph that summarizes the features. You can follow this example, which I've written for my dog Honey. Then, lastly, write a sentence stating what the pet still needs to work on to realize its potential.

> Honey is warm, loving, and loyal (categorical and species codes). He believes in connection, unless separated from his friend Lucky the Labrador (personal, karma). He is communicative (personal, dharma) and has successfully moved through all stages to maturation, which he reflects in his ability to pause and think about his actions (personal, experiences). He exhibits only active traits (personal, personality), loves to move (personal, red coat) and seems very self-aware (personal, brown eyes).

> *Must Work On:* Honey needs to learn how to trust himself even when Lucky isn't around.

7: **Describe Yourself.** Now use the gathered data to analyze yourself in comparison to your pet. Following is my example, which covers all the factors I used with Honey. I also added a conclusion.

> Like Honey, Cyndi is warm, loving, and loyal. She is primarily a connector, unless she feels separated from the Spirit. Like Honey, she is a dharmic communicator and is in the maturation stage, often performing self-assessment and offering care to others. Unlike Honey, she exhibits both active and passive personality traits but shares much of Honey's passion toward life, though she also can be introverted. Like Honey, she is extremely self-aware, but she is also quite mental (yellow hair) and loves data (blue eyes).
>
> *Must Work On:* Cyndi shares several qualities with Honey but needs to work more on her relationship with Spirit while making time for her introversion.

8: **Close.** When ready, ask the Spirit to gently release you from this process. Return to your everyday life.

Now that you have a sense of your pet's energetic signature—and why that pet might be in your life—it's time to jump into the main course of the book and learn all about your pet's energetic system.

Chapter Three
Your Pet's Energy System

> *We are the earth, made of the*
> *same stuff; there is no other, no*
> *division between us and "lower"*
> *or "higher" forms of being.*
>
> Estella Lauder

All of earth is composed of energy, physical and subtle. We alter physical reality by directing subtle energy with our consciousness.

This concept summarizes the theme of this book. The caveat is that we need data and tools if we're to support a pet and pet/human relationship through energetics. Otherwise, altering energy, especially subtle energy, is about as easy as shaping water into the form of a box—or into a pig, for that matter. In this chapter I'll educate you about the subtle systems you'll assess and maneuver to improve your pet's life.

There are three structures within the subtle energy anatomy: centers, channels, and fields. In this chapter I'll discuss all three of these structures with an emphasis on the chakras, the most powerful and accessible of the subtle energy centers. The heavy lifting part of this chapter constitutes an in-depth presentation of the twelve chakras as they appear in and apply to pets. Before sharing this information, which will serve as a go-to reference for the rest of this book, I'll also compare the human chakra system, presented in chapter 1, with a pet's system. This data will make it easier to work with your own structure when working on your pet's.

I'll also exhibit several pet chakra illustrations. The fundamental illustration will showcase the mammalian chakra structure. Additional images will help you locate chakras on other types of natural beings, including birds, arthropods, and reptiles. By the time you're finished with this chapter, you'll be ready to start figuring out what's occurring on the subtle level of your natural friends.

Your Pet's Three Energetic Structures
What Makes Them Tick

You can read a clock, even reset the time, by manipulating a few gadgets. If you need to make a repair or get fancier, you have to understand the clock's underlying mechanics, and so it goes with a pet's chakra system.

This section will delve deeply into two of the main topics featured in chapter 1, which are the subtle anatomy and its usage of light and sound.

The Three Basic Subtle Structures

As already explained, subtle energy is processed through the three main structures of the subtle anatomy. These are the centers, channels, and fields, each of which transforms subtle energy into physical energy and vice versa. The main subtle centers are the chakras, of which there are twelve. Seven are located in the body and affixed in the spine (or the equivalent of the spine), and five are found outside of the body proper, although each of these is also secured in the body. No matter the chakra's location, each regulates a specific set of physical, psychological, and spiritual functions.

But you already knew that. What I haven't explained is the structure of a chakra, a distinction that will become very important when delivering healing through the chakras. Each chakra is actually composed of two wheels, or layers. Both layers hold very different programs. The inner wheels are the more "perfected" in that during preconception, a pet's spirit encodes them with dharmic programming. The outer wheels are scripted by the soul, which loads them with karmic issues, also during preconception. As a pet's life ensues, the outer wheels become the storage houses for newly minted experiences and ideas. These memories, the pet's unconscious conclusions about them, and the imprint of events and interactions are all encoded on the outer wheels of the chakras that they resonate with.

In regard to subtle channels, there are two main types. In the Hindu view of the esoteric anatomy, the major subtle channels are the nadis, which basically equate with the nerves. The most vital nadi runs through the physical spine (or spinal equivalent), and two other important nadis manage the parasympathetic (relaxing) and sympathetic (excitatory) nervous systems. All three nadis also flow through the seven in-body chakras, thus interconnecting the physical and subtle bodies. While we won't directly interact with the nadis, I want you to know that when relating to a chakra, you are substantively altering the central nervous system.

Asian subtle systems also work with subtle energy channels but most frequently call them meridians. For the most part, meridians are different than the nadis in that they are electromagnetic tubules that flow through the connective tissue, passing energy between the connective tissue, cardiovascular system, and central nervous system. The Hindu and Asian systems somewhat intersect in that a handful of meridians and their external entry points, called acupoints, are comparable to specific nadis and chakras. In chapter 7 I'll teach you an easy technique for releasing shock using an acupoint.

As compared to the subtle channels, this book will make more use of the third subtle structure, the auric field. Each of the twelve auric fields is an extension of a chakra. This means that you can interact with a chakra by working its related field, and vice versa. Hence a bit more knowledge about the auric field is in order.

First, I'm going to explain how the chakras generate the auric fields. The energies affecting and generated by the seven in-body chakras twirl in a circular fashion in the front and backside of the body, making them look like vortexes. The whirling energy of these seven chakras eventually forms independent but interlocking bands of subtle energy that encompass the body. Meanwhile, the five out-of-body chakras, which also swirl like whirlpools, generate energies that flow in two primary directions. One arm of the energy anchors in a particular organ in the body and another arm creates an external layer of energy. All twelve bands of energy—the auric fields—are stacked in the order of densest to lightest. As shared in chapter 1, the first auric field is closest to the body. Next is the tenth auric field, and then the second, third, and fourth auric fields, and so on. The eleventh auric field lies over the ninth, and the twelfth follows.

Collectively, the auric layers provide protection and energetic filtering, forming a matrix-like skein called the subtle energy boundary. Taken separately, each field acts like a sieve that lets in and emanates energy based on the programming in its correlated chakra. For instance, imagine that your pet was physically kicked as a tiny puppy. As you'll learn in this chapter, this stage of development is ruled by the first chakra, which governs survival issues. That puppy leaves that stage with a belief stored in its first chakra such as "I deserve to be abused." The first auric field will reflect that negative belief, sending a subtle email into the world that tells anyone and everyone that this dog is available for abuse. Hence that dog, until the negative belief is cleared, could attract people who will kick it or otherwise abuse it. Most likely the dog, knowing it's vulnerable, will also shy away from people, assuming the worst.

We can assess a chakra but also its related field to figure out what is going on with our pet. However, an auric field can also hold positive or negative energies that haven't yet lodged in the corresponding chakra. For instance, the fourth auric field, which relates to the fourth chakra, regulates relationships. Imagine that your pet's fourth auric field has absorbed bits and pieces of an argument you recently had with a family member. Newly entered subtle energy typically lingers for a while in the field before it completely lands in a chakra, where it's harder to clear. If you can clear this energy before it's anchored, you can deter further injury. You'll be shown how to use an acupoint in chapter 7 to do just that.

As implied through the just-shared examples, the energy held within one structure is shared amongst many structures. How exactly does this distribution take place? The answer is light and sound.

It's All About Light and Sound

Energy has two main forms, which are light and sound. Both exist as physical and subtle energies. Thus do the physical and subtle universes flow into and create each other.

Light is formally called electromagnetic radiation, and sound is produced by sonic waves. Like everything in the world, a pet is actually a collection of light and sound waves. On the physical level, every cell and organ pulses with electricity. In turn, electricity produces magnetic and electromagnetic fields, or light. The hormones and other chemicals in the body rely on light to enable organic function. At the same time that every bodily component is shining a light into the universe, it is also emanating sounds. Actually, every cell, organ, and microbe in the body generates its own unique sound, which blends into a wonderful, if unusual, concerto.

On the subtle level, all subtle structures operate on—and emit—their own vibrational frequencies, which also reduce to both light and sound. From one point of view, you could picture these frequencies as bands of light and sound that run horizontally through each chakra from the outside world. Simultaneously, a chakra is generating the same frequencies, which are carried into the world. Every chakra, as well as its correlated auric field, mainly interacts with the colors and tones that match the frequencies of that horizontal band of energy.

In the body, each horizontal band of chakric energy is stacked atop another horizontal band, thus allowing communication between chakras. Chakras aren't closed vehicles. One blends into another. For instance, the first chakra is red and the second chakra is orange. This means that there are various shades of red-orange hues between them. What's on the other side of the orange chakra? Why, orange-yellow bands that stair-step to the yellow chakra. Even the chakras outside of the body communicate, as each locks into the physical body, thus participating in the dance of light and sound. A similar passing of communication occurs between auric fields as one field flows into the other. And in the same way that chakras pass information between themselves and their correlated auric fields, the meridians and nadis also share data amongst themselves and with their fellow subtle structures.

The only difference between the light and sound—or messages—generated by the physical versus subtle structures is measurability. The frequencies of the body are perceived through our five senses, whereas subtle energies are too fast or slow to easily hear, see, sense, smell, or feel. Chakras to the rescue! As I've stated already, chakras can transform physical energy into subtle energy and vice versa. This means that chakras can change subtle messages into physical communications that the brain can understand. This spiritual (or psychic and intuitive) function is performed by every chakra. For instance, the second chakra, which processes emotional data, will help you feel others' feelings in your body. It will also send psychic impressions of your feelings into the world. The fifth chakra, which is verbal in nature, will enable you to receive clairaudient information, turn it into words in your head, and dispatch the same to others.

In general, the lower a subtle structure is in relationship to the body—or the closer it is to the body—the lower its frequencies. The opposite is also true. The subtle structures that are higher up in the body are higher in frequency. Lower-frequency energies create the strongest effect in dense or physical reality. Higher-frequency energies are the most spiritual. And what about frequencies in the mid range? These affect the material and spiritual universes, and for this reason I consider them psychological in nature. I'll more fully explain how to apply this knowledge for pet care as this book proceeds.

While energetic experts frequently use techniques involving light and sound to work on humans, it's especially important to do this for pets because they enjoy a more expanded range of both than we do.

The Subtle Light and Sound of Your Pet

We can create more powerful change through subtle interactions with pets than with humans because pets are even more subtly sensitive. In other words, pets can access lights and sounds that are subtle to humans but normal to them.

The truth is that we humans actually perceive very little of the light and sound manufactured in our bodies or available in the environment. In fact, our eyes can only see about .0035 percent of the electromagnetic spectrum measured on a linear scale, and about 2.3 percent of all visible light (Link 2007). Of all sounds, humans can only hear about one-fifth of all frequencies (Akpan 2015).

Members of the nonhuman nations aren't nearly as limited. Mammals including dogs, cats, rodents, and ferrets can see ultraviolet light, which is higher in frequency than visible light. Same with many species of birds, reptiles, insects, and fishes, some of which, like snakes, can also perceive infrared frequencies, which are lower in frequency than visible light (Aktipis 2015).

Many natural beings also hear frequencies that humans cannot. The average human ear can perceive sounds between 20 and 20,000 hertz. Dogs can hear frequencies twice that of humans and make out noises that are four times farther away. Cats hear even better than their doggie mates (Wonderopolis, n.d.). Insects have tympanal organs that are far more sensitive than human ears, while spiders and cockroaches have tiny leg hairs that pick up sounds. Even though fish don't have physical ears, perceiving sounds through lateral lines—and, for some, earlike brain structures—they can pick up on sounds that we can't (Dodero Hearing Center 2013).

The conclusion is that many members of the nonhuman nations function on energies that are subtle to humans. This means that we must employ subtle knowledge if we're to truly aid our pets, especially concentrating on light and sound. With this in mind, the rest of this chapter is devoted to teaching you about your pet's subtle anatomy, highlighting the chakras, the core subtle units for light and sound.

Your Pet's Chakra System
A Comparative Analysis

All natural beings have a twelve-chakra system, including humans and pets. You were first introduced to the human chakras in chapter 1; these were illustrated in figure 1. You were also shown mammalian chakras on figures 2 and 3. Keep these illustrations in mind as I discuss a few of the differences between a pet's and a human's chakra system before I more thoroughly describe all twelve pet chakras. This comparative analysis will assist you in working through your own chakra-based issues if they arise when you're interacting with a pet's chakras.

In a nutshell, most esoteric pet experts believe that the seven in-body chakras of humans and pets are similar in function. These seven chakras lock into the spine, if a pet has a spine. If not, they are centered in the middle of the body. Each of the seven in-body chakras also interacts with a specific endocrine gland, or the parts of a pet's body that perform endocrine functions, and manages its own set of physical, psychological, and spiritual functions. Succinctly, the seven in-body chakras of a pet manage the same general functions that they accomplish in a human:

> **First Chakra:** survival
>
> **Second Chakra:** emotions

Third Chakra: mentality

Fourth Chakra: relationship

Fifth Chakra: communication

Sixth Chakra: vision

Seventh Chakra: spirituality

A pet's five out-of-body chakras are also similar in function to those found in a person. As do their in-body kin, each of these centers manages an endocrine gland and also a set of physical, psychological, and spiritual concerns. However, there are a few pet-specific distinctions in these chakras that make them different than those in humans.

First of all, the basic duties of each of these five out-of-body chakras, which are similar to the jobs performed in humans, are as follows.

Eighth: mysticism

Ninth: harmonizing

Tenth: elemental and environmental connections

Bud Chakras: attune to environmental vibrations and changes (officially part of the tenth chakra)

Eleventh: command of forces

Twelfth: unique; reflects dharma and conveys a special spiritual gift

As in humans, the major endocrine gland associated with the eighth chakra is the thymus. But there is an additional bodily location in mammals, rodents, and members of many other nonhuman nations. This is the brachial or key chakra, which is found in the shoulder area in natural beings with shoulders. Lying atop both shoulder blades, this eighth chakra access point transforms the shoulders into a communication vehicle between pets and people. Because the eighth chakra links beings to various planes of existence, a pet's shoulder area can actually enable energetic exchanges between human and pet souls across time.

As in humans, a pet's ninth chakra is above the head and is secured in the breathing system. It manages a pet's ability to harmonize with others. A pet's tenth chakra, like a human's, is found under the feet and is moored in the earth but is also uniquely linked to the bud chakras, a term used by esoteric pet professionals.

Bud chakras are found on the underside of a pet's pad, paw, hoof, claw, or related area, and also at the base of a pet's ear or hearing apparatus. Their job is to sense changes in the environment, such as in the weather, and connect a living being to the natural world. Through the ear location, a pet can "hear" vibrations that are so subtle that they don't make noise. The bud chakra is also found on the tips of a bird's wings or a fish's fins.

Rounding out the chakra system, a pet's eleventh chakra is woven through their muscles and connective tissue and has the same function as it does in humans, which is to enable the command of natural and supernatural forces. As you can see on figure 1, the eleventh chakra is focused in the hands and feet in humans. In pets, the apparatus of movement belongs to their tenth chakra, although the eleventh chakra operates the muscles that make these body parts (like feet or claws) work. And last but not least, the twelfth chakra in both non-human and human nations is positioned at the outer bounds of the auric field and is unique to each being. In natural beings, the twelfth chakra anchors into twenty-one minor sites.

These sites are secondary chakras, and they appear in pets as structures supporting specific bodily areas, if a pet has these areas. They are found on places like the nose, tail, and ears. I describe them on page 89's chart called "A Pet's Twenty-One Secondary Chakras."

What's in a Chakra?

In order to really decipher and access your pet's chakra system, however, you'll need a lot more information than what I've just provided. The in-depth synopsis of each chakra will cover the following functions:

Chakra Name: Will be listed numerically. The seven in-body chakras will also be labeled with their Sanskrit name, the language first used to depict chakras in the Hindu nation.

Location: General physical area hosting the chakra. If dealing with an out-of-body chakra, I'll share its externalized location and also its in-body anchor point.

Purpose: A summative word or phrase depicting the chakra's tasks.

Color: The color of the vibrational band of frequencies that a chakra operates on and emanates.

Physical Jobs: Examples of the bodily structures and functions performed by the chakra. We'll feature the symptoms of a chakric problem in the next chapter.

Psychological Functions: The emotional and mental functions of the chakra.

Spiritual Abilities: Each chakra is a lens for a specific type of psychic knowledge or intuitive function, which is labeled and described.

Stage Activation: A chakra is fully awakened or activated at a distinct stage. Stages were introduced in chapter 2's section called "Your Pet's This-Life Experiences," and I include reminders in the following list. This information can help you track physical, psychological, and spiritual issues to a chakra and figure out the stage at which a problem incurred. This knowledge can make it easier to understand a problem and arrive at the best solution.

The number signifying a stage is different than the chakra number. Because this can be confusing, I'm providing a cheat sheet that describes each stage with its numerical label, a one- or two-word tag, and the correlated chakra. I'll drop this information into the upcoming chakra descriptions.

CHART: *A Pet's Stages of Development*

Stage	Keywords	Chakra
First	Dharmic Selection	Ninth
Second	Karmic Selection	Eighth
Third	Programming	Tenth
Fourth	Survival	First
Fifth	Socialization	Second
Sixth	Learning	Third
Seventh	Relating	Fourth
Eighth	Communication	Fifth

Stage	Keywords	Chakra
Ninth	Self-Awareness	Sixth
Tenth	Spiritualization	Seventh
Eleventh	Supernatural Power	Eleventh
Twelfth	Transformational	Twelfth

Element: Most chakras process one or two specific elements, which are the natural building blocks of everything on earth and in the cosmos. I work with a twelve-element system, and in the chakra descriptions, I will attribute at least one element to each chakra. I'll also describe each element. This information is based on my own perception and data culled from several cultures.

Sound: In the Hindu system, chakras are affiliated with a major sound, which can tonify that chakra. I'll share the Hindu sound affiliated with the seven in-body chakras and my own ideas about the additional five chakric sounds. Regarding the latter, I employ a Sanskrit sound or term that reflects the meaning of the chakra. I'll provide the sound and its meaning.

Related Auric Field: Every chakra generates an auric field. In the chakra descriptions, I'll name the field, tell you where it is located outside of the body, and describe its major tasks. Refer to figure 4 to discover the location of a pet's auric fields. Figure 3 also showcases a mammal's chakras, which are the sole subject of figures 2 and 3. Figure 5 depicts a human's auric field, allowing you to compare it with the fields of a pet in figure 4.

Auric Field	Color
1	red
2	orange
3	yellow
4	green
5	blue
6	violet
7	white
8	black or silver
9	gold
10	brown
11	pink
12	clear

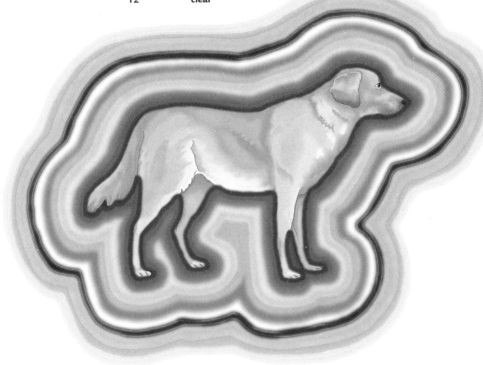

Figure 4: A Pet's Auric Field

Both humans and pets have an auric field composed of twelve
individual fields. The first field begins closest to the body.

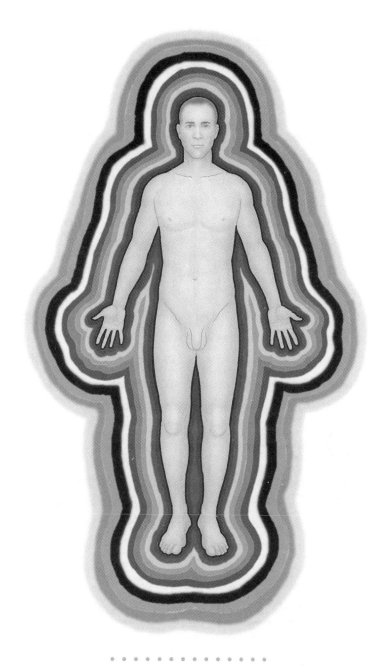

Figure 5: A Human's Auric Field

The first field is located next to the body; the twelfth is farthest away.

First Chakra: Muladhara

Location: Base of spine or area functioning as the spine

Purpose: Physicality and survival

Color: Red

Physical Jobs: Assures survival. Runs areas and organs comparable to adrenals, hips, reproductive organs, skin, lower orifices, and excretory system. In a pet with fur, scales, feathers, and the like, a malady encompassing most of these coverings is considered first chakra, although if a foot or hand-like area is involved, you'll also examine the tenth chakra.

Psychological Functions: Feelings and beliefs regarding survival and security, such as believing that the self deserves to exist.

Spiritual Abilities: Physical empathy, which is the ability to sense another's physical sensations or illness in one's own body. The pet also can send bodily sensations to others through this ability.

Stage Activation: Survival. Involves the transference of parental issues during in utero and infancy to assure survival.

Element: Fire, representing passion, movement, and vitality

Sound: *Lam*

Related Auric Field: The first auric field is inside and right outside of the skin. It attracts events and beings that will help guarantee survival and grant security, sending messages into the world to draw safe people, beings, and events to the self.

Second Chakra: Svadhisthana

Location: In abdomen or related area

Purpose: Emotions and creativity

Color: Orange

Physical Jobs: Governs digestive functions. Manages physical sites comparable to the small intestine, ovaries, testes, and sacral vertebrae.

Psychological Functions: Feelings and beliefs related to bonding, creativity, and the relationship between self and others, as well as sensuality and liveliness.

Spiritual Abilities: Feeling empathy, which involves sensing others' feelings within the self and conveying one's feelings to others.

Stage Activation: Socialization. Encoded during early childhood, this skill is affected by how the pet relates to members of its bio-family and surrounding natural beings or persons.

Element: Water, which relates to intuitive and emotional flow

Sound: *Vam*

Related Auric Field: The second field is outside of the tenth field. It disseminates a pet's feelings into the world and brings in others' feelings.

Third Chakra: Manipura

Location: Solar plexus or stomach region

Purpose: Mentality and willpower

Color: Yellow

Physical Jobs: Manages digestive processes and the organs involved, such as the liver, stomach, spleen, gallbladder, kidneys, and more, as well as the middle of the spine.

Psychological Functions: This chakra is the basin for thoughts and beliefs that form judgments, opinions, and actions/behaviors related to self-esteem, self-confidence, and the relationship with power.

Spiritual Abilities: Mental empathy, also called claircognizance, which is the ability to sense others' attitudes and beliefs and send the same into the world.

Stage Activation: Learning. Activated in early maturity, during this stage a pet demonstrates what it has learned and if it can follow others' directives.

Element: Wood, which supports goals, life changes, and positive life habits; also the element of air, which relates to the transmission of ideas and ideals.

Sound: *Ram*

Related Auric Field: This field lies outside of the second field. It sends a pet's thoughts and opinions into the world and brings in the same from others.

Fourth Chakra: Anahata

Location: Heart or chest area

Purpose: Love, relationship, and healing

Color: Green

Physical Jobs: Runs cardiovascular/circulatory system, lungs, breasts, shoulders, ribs, chest, and arms. Also regulates the functions of the cardiac vertebrae or related area.

Psychological Functions: Manages higher emotions and virtues, allowing the giving and taking of love and healing.

Spiritual Abilities: Relational empathy, which invites knowledge of others' higher emotional, relational, and healing needs and sends the same information from the pet into the world.

Stage Activation: Relating. Occurring during early maturity, at this stage the pet's soul leans toward being more karmic, or working through past issues, or dharmic, which involves making strides in its purpose and understanding of love.

Element: Star, which is a combination of fire and ether. Star blends passion with the Spirit's higher ideals. This is the perfect element for the heart, which lies in the center of the in-body chakra system. Star energy merges fire from the first chakra with ether from the seventh chakra.

Sound: *Yam*

Related Auric Field: The fourth field lies outside the third field. It attracts love and healing and allows the same to be sent to others.

Fifth Chakra: Vishuddha

Location: Throat area

Purpose: Communication and expression

Color: Blue

Physical Jobs: Regulates the throat, jaws, teeth, mouth, thyroid, esophagus, neck, and cervical vertebrae, or whichever bodily parts serve these functions.

Psychological Functions: Governs beliefs related to communication, such as a pet's sense of responsibility, ability to say yes or no, and willingness to receive guidance.

Spiritual Abilities: Verbal empathy, which is the ability to psychically hear and emanate auditory guidance in the language or expression related to the pet.

Stage Activation: Communicating. During early maturity, a pet displays its ability to express its needs and respond to others' verbal commands or desires.

Element: Sound, which conveys messages related to power.

Sound: *Ham*

Related Auric Field: The fifth field, found outside of the fourth field, ushers in spiritual guidance, others' telepathic thoughts and verbalizations, and sends psychically packed auditory messages into the world.

Sixth Chakra: Ajna

Location: Brow or area near eyes

Purpose: Vision and perception

Color: Violet

Physical Jobs: Manages the lower part of the brain and upper spinal area, organs associated with sight, and the brain's major hormone gland, which in mammals is the pituitary.

Psychological Functions: Herein lies the ability to perceive truth, especially about the self.

Spiritual Abilities: Visual empathy, also called clairvoyance, which is the ability to receive and send psychic images.

Stage Activation: Self-awareness. Activates during middle maturity to reveal a pet's self-image. At this stage, a pet frequently mirrors the often hidden self-image of a human companion.

Element: Light, the spectrum of subtle energies that express love.

Sound: *Om*

Related Auric Field: The sixth field, which lies outside of the fifth field, sends psychic pictures of a pet's self-image, needs, and thoughts into the world. It also brings in psychic impressions with the same meaning from others.

Seventh Chakra: Sahasrara

Location: Top of the head or brain region

Purpose: Spirituality and higher thinking

Color: White

Physical Jobs: Manages the parts of brain associated with higher thinking, consciousness, sleeping, and mood. In many pets, it governs the pineal gland, cerebral cavity, cerebral plexus, and cranium, or similar bodily parts.

Psychological Functions: Responds to higher virtues such as truth, hope, and love.

Spiritual Abilities: Spiritual empathy, also called prophecy, allows a pet to understand the positive and negative energies of others, and to reflect—or respond to—another's true spiritual nature.

Stage Activation: Spiritualization. During late maturity, a pet's karma can smooth out and its empathic nature can emerge, along with its dharmic ability to reflect spiritual ideals.

Element: Ether, which reflects the consciousness of the Spirit, allows a pet to display higher virtues and principles.

Sound: *Om*

Related Auric Field: The seventh field lies atop the sixth field. It detects negativity and positivity while sending spiritual messages into the world.

Eighth Chakra

Location: Two inches above the head and anchored in the thymus or equivalent immune regulator; also found in shoulder blade region.

Purpose: Mysticism, shamanism, and karma

Color: Black or silver; black absorbs energy to use as power, and silver deflects negativity and produces love. The colors vary based on the pet's personality.

Physical Jobs: Regulates immune processes, potentially causing (or curing) autoimmune disorders and chronic illnesses.

Psychological Functions: The eighth chakra connects to the past, the present, and possible futures, also storing all karmic issues and resolutions. It is the home of the Akashic Records, the library of a pet's activities and reflections across time, as well as other types of spiritual records.

Spiritual Abilities: Mystical empathy. Basically, the eighth chakra invites the shamanic use of all spiritual abilities and powers in accessing energies and beings across time.

Stage Activation: Karmic selection. During preconception, the pet's soul works with its spiritual guides to decide what karma will be encoded in the genes and epigenes. This means that a pet soul's eighth chakra powers, often employed in past lives, are available throughout a pet's life.

Element: Metal, which deflects negativity and allows the transmission of shamanic information and messages from the Spirit and inter-dimensional beings.

Sound: *Akasha*, which means "sky" and describes the information stored in the Akashic Records.

Related Auric Field: The eighth field, outside of the seventh field, accesses all time and space, forging links with beings and energies across dimensions. It "decides" what communications to generate or receive based on soul issues, or karma.

Ninth Chakra

Location: About two feet over the head, anchored in the breathing apparatus.

Purpose: Harmonizing

Color: Gold

Physical Jobs: Manages diaphragm or related breathing apparatus and mechanisms.

Psychological Functions: Represents the highest aspects of the soul, enabling it to harmonize with others' souls and higher ideals.

Spiritual Abilities: Harmonic empathy, the ability to deeply resonate with others.

Stage Activation: Dharmic selection, which occurs during preconception. During this stage, the pet's spirit selects the dharma that will be encrypted in the future embryo's genes and epigenetics.

Element: Star, a blend of ether, which reflects heavenly principles, and fire, the energy of passion.

Sound: *Samata* or "evenness," the condition of harmony.

Related Auric Field: The ninth auric field is outside of the eighth field. The ninth field attracts and disseminates energy that will create harmony and peace.

Tenth Chakra

Location: About two feet underneath the feet or the body part low to the ground; in pets, also associated with the bud chakras, which are located on body parts equivalent to the feet/hands/paws and the area under the ear opening.

Purpose: Groundedness and relationship to the environment.

Color: Brown

Physical Jobs: Manages the bones, stem cells, genes, and epigenetics, as well as the legs, feet, and underneath the ears or equivalent body parts, including parts of the ear area that invite attunement to the environment. If a condition on the skin or equivalent of fur, feathers, or gills also includes the equivalency of the feet or hands, it will involve the first and tenth chakras.

Psychological Functions: This chakra reflects a pet's sense of self in the environment.

Spiritual Abilities: Environmental empathy, the ability to be aware of and sense what is, has, or will occur in the environment and amongst the elements.

Stage Activation: Programming, which occurs at conception. The codes of the soul and spirit are imprinted in the genes and epigenetics of the emerging embryo, seeding karmic and dharmic programs. These imprints will determine the pet's relationship with their environment and surroundings.

Element: Earth, which is grounded, warm, and enables growth; also stone, which stores the history of an area. This history includes the stories of a habitat and the beings that have dwelled upon it.

Sound: *Ahimsa*, which reflects the belief in nonviolence and respect for all.

Related Auric Field: The tenth auric field is right outside of the first field. It is also called the etheric layer and mirrors all of a pet's karmic and dharmic programming, genetic and epigenetic patterning, and brings in energies needed to heal or balance karmic and dharmic programming. It also sends out messages to attract other pets, people, or events to help accomplish the pet's spiritual goals.

Eleventh Chakra

Location: Located in the eleventh auric field, locking into the body through the connective tissue and muscles.

Purpose: Commanding of forces; supernatural connection to forces—light, dark, environmental, and cosmic. Can influence bud chakras to "perform" supernatural actions.

Color: Rose

Physical Jobs: Basically runs the muscles and connective tissue, thereby enabling the locomotion of the tenth chakra's bud chakras.

Psychological Functions: Relates to beliefs about the ability to steer the natural and supernatural forces of the world.

Spiritual Abilities: Force empathy, which is the ability to sense and command natural and supernatural forces. These forces can be good or bad; environmental, such as involving weather, elements, or natural beings; and cosmic, either paranormal or heavenly.

Stage Activation: Supernatural power. Most strongly illuminated during early to mid-decline, during which time supernatural abilities might emerge as the body fades.

Element: Star, which combines fire and ether.

Sound: *Seva,* which means "service."

Related Auric Field: The eleventh field surrounds the ninth. It sends the pet's directives into the world to stir natural and supernatural responses and attracts forces the pet can command.

Twelfth Chakra

Location: In the twelfth auric field, connecting into the body through the minor chakras, which are outlined in the chart on page 89.

Purpose: This chakra's overall job differs from pet to pet, as it reflects the pet's very unique spiritual self.

Color: Clear or translucent

Physical Jobs: Through the personal spirit of the pet, the chakra manages the secondary organs and chakras of the pet's body.

Psychological Functions: These are personal to the pet in that they are reflective of their relationship with the Spirit.

Spiritual Abilities: These are personal to the pet but reflect a power unique and special to their spirit, such as the ability to create happy endings or help humans remember their true nature.

Stage Activation: Transformation, which occurs when the pet is declining, dying, and entering the afterlife. Allows for the true presentation of the pet's nature; reveals what the pet has or hasn't worked through karmically; and showcases the pet's authentic dharmic essence.

Element: Presence. This element is representative of the perfection of the Spirit made personal to the pet.

Sound: *Aham*, which means "I." I chose this term because the twelfth chakra is the outer boundary of a pet's true self.

Related Auric Field: The twelfth auric field is outside of the eleventh and all other auric fields. It brings in energies needed to support the pet's unique gift and sends the energies of this gift into the world and beyond.

Want to see what the twelve chakras look like in pets? I've created the following illustrations to help you do so. These are partially based on information available from energy experts who have developed chakra illustrations for dogs, cats, horses, reptiles, fish, birds, guinea pigs, hamsters, and rabbits. Unlike my images, these feature seven rather than twelve chakras. You can easily find the various seven-chakra pet systems by doing an internet search of "chakras" and the type of pet from the list I just provided. To fill in the gap between what is known and unknown about pet chakras, I have supplemented the available material with insights from my intuition and experience.

Figures 6 and 7 depict avian chakras; figure 8 uses a lizard illustration to reveal the chakras of most reptiles and amphibians; figure 9 illustrates fish; figure 10 portrays a spider and also other invertebrates; and figure 11 simultaneously shows the chakras of a snake and conveys the magical caduceus, the staff of enlightenment often used to symbolize the power of the chakras.

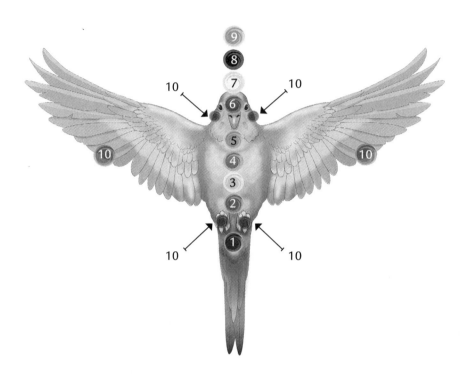

Figure 6: Bird Chakras' Front View

This frontal view of a bird depicts the location of ten of their twelve chakras.
A bird's tenth chakra, which includes the bud chakras, lies underneath
the claws and near the ear fissures, and includes the windtips.

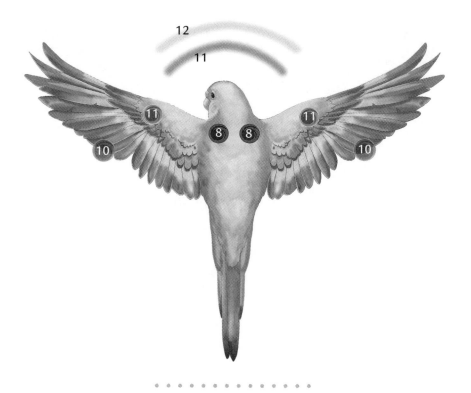

Figure 7: Bird Chakras' Back View

This back view of a bird shows the shoulder blade region associated with
the eighth chakra and the locations of the eleventh and twelfth chakras. The
eleventh is outside of the body as well as linked with the bird's muscles.

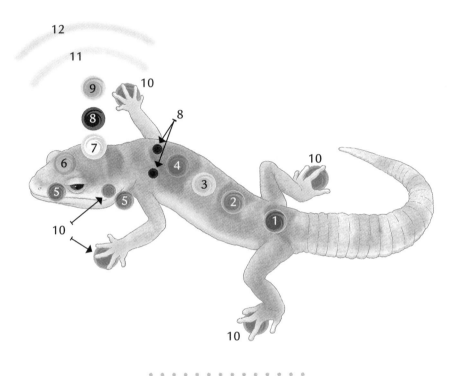

Figure 8: Lizard and Other Reptilian Chakras

This shows a lizard's twelve chakras and is representative of other reptiles and most amphibians. Because they are vertebrates, the chakras in reptiles and amphibians are similar in location to those found in mammals.

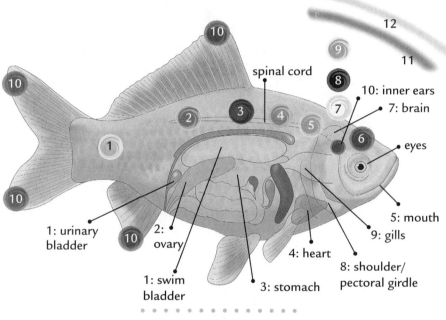

Figure 9: Fish Chakras

Several organs are labeled to help you locate the chakras. Some of them are labeled with the chakra and some are independent of the chakras. In a fish, there are three parts to the tenth chakra: the fins (for locomotion), the inner ears or internal bones (to assess noise), and the lateral lines (these react to vibrations). The bud chakras, part of the tenth chakra, are most associated with fins.

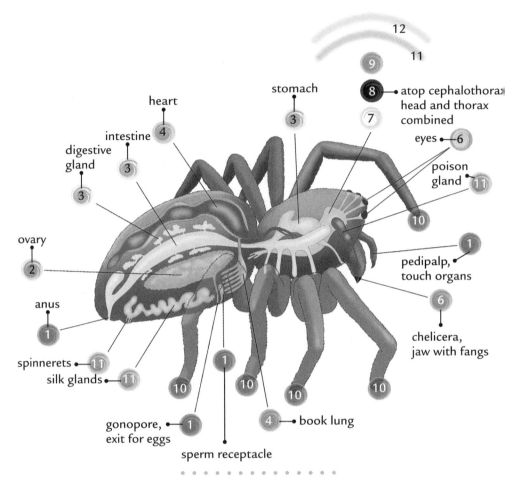

Figure 10: Chakras in Spiders and Other Invertebrates

The chakras of spiders and other invertebrates are hard to locate. Because of this, the chakras are labeled in association with their main organs. The legs are part of a spider's tenth chakra, the ends of which constitute the bud chakras. The eleventh chakra, which allows a spider to command forces through the production of venom and silk, includes bodily areas such as the spinnerets, silk glands, and poison gland.

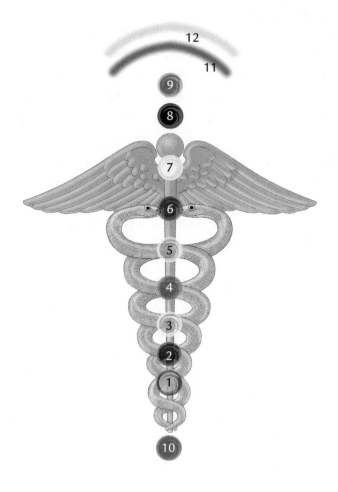

Figure 11: Chakras in a Snake

This illustration shows the location of a snake's chakras upon a
caduceus, the symbol of medicine. The staff represents the sushumna
nadi and the two snakes characterize the ida and pingala nadis, which
are explained in this chapter. Shown are all twelve chakras. The bud
chakras, part of the tenth chakra, comprise the entire underbelly.

Secondary Chakras

Pets can have up to twenty-one secondary chakras, which are extensions of the twelfth chakra, which is interwoven within the twelfth auric field. If a pet lacks a body part, it won't have the corresponding secondary chakra. Secondary chakras are also called minor chakras. They form smaller vortexes than do the major chakras and are often associated with a bodily intersection, such as a joint.

While many energy experts suggest that there are twenty-one secondary chakras, I have yet to find a full listing. I have conducted research to figure out which of the many points on a pet's body would qualify as a secondary chakra. The research includes data from Hindu philosophies, Taoism, Ayurveda, animal experts, and other sources. But you have to "hang loose" when analyzing a pet for minor chakras. For instance, let's consider the knees.

Some people believe that mammals have either four knees or four elbows or a mix of both. Actually, cats functionally have knees on their back legs and elbows on the front, as per the comparison to humans. It's the same with dogs, horses, and rodents. Spiders have forty-eight knees. Birds have knees that bend the same as do human knees, and ants have fifty-six knees. Snakes have none.

How about the eyes, a commonplace secondary chakra? All vertebrates have two eyes, but arachnids can have up to eight eyes. A praying mantis might employ five eyes. If you own a starfish pet, which we don't address in this book, know that your pet has an eye at the end of each arm.

And how about that secondary nose chakra? It's easy to spot the nose chakra on a mammal or rodent, but the appearance of the olfactory organs differs in other pets. Spiders are one of the few arthropods that can smell. To do this, they use a hair-like structure located around the legs. Fish have little holes called nares, which open to an inner chamber lined with sensory pads. And snakes smell with organs on the roof of their mouths. Smell is the oldest known sense and alerts pets to danger or what they desire, but the apparatus can differ.

With these caveats in mind, the following chart presents pets' secondary chakras and describes their energetic functions. No matter how much physical area is covered by a single chakra—i.e., there are two eyes and a pet can have dozens of whiskers—it adds up to a single chakra. I use labels here that are the most familiar in humans. You can simply substitute the correct terms for your pet's similar body part. For instance, a pet's top of foot might be the top of a claw or paw.

CHART: *A Pet's Twenty-One Secondary Chakras*

Secondary Chakra	Energetic Function
Knees	Provide flexibility and direction.
Nose	On the tip of the nose, this chakra senses physical and subtle olfactory information. It is often psychically seen as gray or shiny silver.
Elbows	Elbows represent the ability to move freely and make radical change when needed.
Eyes	Eyes are the gateway to the soul and psychically represent intelligence, light, clairvoyance, and morality.
Tips of the Ears	The tip of a pet's ear covering, like a dog's earflap, hosts a minor chakra that enables clairaudient hearing. Fish have lateral lines on their bodies laden with neuroblasts, or primative nerve cells, that "hear" vibrational changes in water pressure. (This chakra isn't the same as the bud chakra, which is located at the base of the ear entrance, such as under a dog's earflap.)
Tip of Tail	Senses danger, love, and the moods of beings in the environment. I believe that pets communicate their needs and moods and can connect into other dimensions through their tails.
Whiskers	Whiskers enable the reading of others' moods and help with navigation. Pets with whiskers can detect the "luckiest" or most fortuitous choices. Whiskers can also be equated with psychic antennae.
Base of Tongue	This chakra enables a pet to find food and detect danger.
Hip Bones	Picks up on others' emotions, sexual desires, and ways to prosper the self.
Ming-men Doorway	An energetic opening between the kidneys that brings in spiritual blessings and the life energy of the ancestors.
Perineum	Gate of life and death; dark entities can enter, but so can additional parts of a pet's soul.
Top of Foot	Grounds a pet in the present moment while allowing changes in direction or goals.

Secondary Chakra	Energetic Function
Top of Shoulders	Distinct from the eighth chakra shoulder blades, the shoulder blade tips reflect burdens happily or unhappily carried.
Armpits	Reflect thoughts and emotions about acceptance by the clan and human companions.
Back of Head (between cranium and cervical vertebrae)	Acts as a doorway for spiritual energy and guidance.
Finger/Toe Joints	Reflect the ability to give and receive; also to hold ground or give way when something undesirable is occurring.
Cranial Bones (or shells around the body, such as on a turtle)	Ability to be spiritually protected while opening to guidance and incoming knowledge.
Wrists/Ankles	Capacity to start and complete.
Jaw Joints	Reflect emotional tension or ease and the ability to "devour" what one wants from life.
Teeth	Each tooth represents a different meridian and a higher truth.
Ribs	Picks up on safety of love—is it safe to love another or not?

Now that you are more knowledgeable about your pet's energetic system, you are ready to acquire a vital bonding tool and learn how to communicate with your pet. You'll make use of this skill when problem-solving for your pet's concerns.

Chapter Four

Pet Communication: The Fundamental Connection

An animal's eyes have the power
to speak a great language.

Martin Buber

What's your pet trying to communicate to you? Do you need to get a message to your pet? In this chapter I'll discuss and demonstrate ways to intuitively communicate with a pet, either directly or through a spiritual guide. Yes, pets have guides, a concept I'll explore in this chapter.

Pet communication is a necessary skill for the human who yearns to support their pet and improve their pet/human bond. You can use this process to analyze for issues, arrive at possible solutions, share information, and just plain enjoy each other's company. Think about how much your pet wants to share with you—and vice versa.

This chapter kicks off with descriptions of the four main intuitive styles that organize the different chakra gifts.

- physical
- spiritual
- verbal
- visual

There is also a "catch-all" style called mystical intuition that enables you to merge all four basic intuitive styles.

A few words of advice will help you pinpoint the style that might work best with your particular pet. Finally, you'll apply Spirit-to-Spirit and another process called Healing Streams of Grace to actually communicate with—and assist—your pet. You'll discover that the latter technique can help you accomplish nearly any pet-related goal, which is why you'll be employing it throughout the remainder of this book.

Ready to communicate? Your pet sure is!

The Four Main Styles of Pet Communication

There are twelve chakra-based intuitive faculties, and each is distinct. These intuitive facilities were first explored in the chakra descriptions in chapter 3 under the heading "Spiritual Abilities." I organize the gifts linked to chakras one to eleven in four categorical styles, also adding a fifth, or combination, style. These categories are physical, spiritual, verbal, and visual intuition, to which we add mystical intuition. The gift associated with the twelfth chakra is unique to each being and therefore can't be categorized.

I like organizing the eleven major intuitive faculties in categories because it is an easy way to remember and access them. And if your pet is adept at one of the chakric gifts in a collection, it usually excels at the others in the grouping. In the exercise in this chapter, which will help you intuitively communicate with your pet, you'll be encouraged to employ an entire grouping but also reduce your intuitive communications to a single chakra, making it easier to focus.

What makes a pet better at one particular intuitive style rather than others? One determinant is a pet's species. As you'll learn in this chapter, certain species are oriented toward interacting through a specific categorical or chakra style rather than others. For instance, snakes are very physical. You can reach them through the physical empathy category and even more specifically through their first chakra. Most fish also fit into the physical empathy category but are more emotional than you might think, and therefore employ their second chakra when intuitively communicating. But a pet's particular personality, noted by their overarching energetic signature, might turn it into a horse of a different color—one horse might be mystical and another entirely physical. Later in this chapter, I'll provide clues for figuring out your particular pet's intuitive abilities.

Before jumping into my descriptions of the individual gifts as per their categorical groupings, I want to define intuition. To me, intuition is the mindful management of subtle energy. Our pets are constantly interacting on the subtle level, directing data at you while picking up messages from you. Most likely, you've been relatively unaware of exactly how much intuitive communicating is already occurring between you and your pet. Understanding the four main intuitive groupings and the chakra gifts within them might strike a chord, helping you realize both how communicative you and your pet already are and can be. Following is a synopsis of the overarching gifts and their chakric subtypes.

Physical Intuition

Physical intuitives sense subtle energy empathically, or in their bodies. There are four subdivisions within this style:

> **Environmental Empathy (Tenth Chakra):** Environmental empaths physically attune to occurrences in their surroundings, the cosmos, the natural environment, and other natural beings. They can also generate subtle energies that can impact the natural world.

> **Physical Empathy (First Chakra):** Physical empaths feel others' bodily sensations in their own body, sometimes even smelling or tasting what another is experiencing. They can also send their own physical sensations into others' bodies.

> **Emotional Empathy (Second Chakra):** Emotional empaths sense others' feelings in their own body and send their feelings into others.

> **Mental Empathy (Third Chakra):** Mental empaths are aware of others' thoughts, beliefs, and motivations, and can send the same to others.

Spiritual Intuition

Plain and simple, spiritual empaths are spiritually aware. They process higher, consciousness-based data in the following ways:

> **Relational Empathy (Fourth Chakra):** Relational empaths can "read" another's need for love, relationship, and healing. They can also disseminate information about their own needs for love and healing.

Spiritual Empathy (Seventh Chakra): Spiritual empaths comprehend others' spiritual purpose, values, and integrity, and also communicate data about their own spiritual personality to others.

Harmonic Empathy (Ninth Chakra): Harmonic empaths sense the discord in others and know how to enable more harmony. They can also share their deepest desires for connection to others.

Force Empathy (Eleventh Chakra): A force empath intuitively senses which supernatural and natural forces are negatively or positively affecting themselves and others. They can also summon and direct forces and sense what another being is doing with the forces at their command. Supernatural forces are magical and invisible. They make instantaneous differences in the physical world. On the other hand, natural forces are composed of elemental properties, such as water, air, wood, and fire. Their effects often seem more commonplace than those produced by supernatural forces.

Verbal Intuition

Verbal intuitives use their fifth chakra to receive and send psychic messages that are auditory in nature. These messages might be physically audible or heard internally, but they can be composed of any verbal medium, including words, writing, songs, sounds, chants, and noises. The difference between a psychically verbal message and an everyday one is that there is a hidden psychic message in the audible sounds or the written phrases.

Visual Intuition

Visual intuitives employ their sixth chakra to receive and send psychic or clairvoyant visualizations. They might see these images on their inner mind screen or through their eyes, but the true meaning of the image is conveyed psychically. Psychic pictures often appear as colors, shapes, symbols, or even movie-like dramatizations. What is an example of an externally conveyed visual message? Imagine that your pet stands near a street sign that showcases what the pet is communicating.

Mystical Intuition

Whether they belong to the human or nonhuman nations, mystical intuitives are shamans, "priest-healers" that can employ any chakra and form of intuition to receive and send subtle information. Shamans can access every subtle and physical realm of existence, conduct interdimensional travel, and connect with spirits from anywhere.

How can you put this information to work? Let's take a look.

The Intuitive Styles in Action

When performing pet communication, you'll usually want to mirror your pet's main intuitive style. They can't easily participate in human language, so you have to use their lingo. To accomplish this goal, I'll further embellish each of the styles and their related chakric gifts to describe how a pet sends subtle data and how you can reply. Of course, you can reverse the process and reach out first!

Physical Intuition

In general, a physically intuitive pet will send a missive to you through the environment or straight into your body. You might touch something they've been holding and receive a bodily sensation or sense their physical, emotional, or mental condition as if it's your own. Environmentally, they might knock a plant off a stand, perhaps insinuating that it needs watering or is poisonous. Specifics are as follows:

> **Environmental Empathy:** Tenth chakra empaths respond to the natural and surrounding world, interacting with objects, such as stones and couches; the eco-habitat, such as plants and trees; the cosmos, such as the sun and stars; and other natural beings, including their fellow pets or wild creatures. To send you a message, an environmentally based pet might set a stone in your lap, act disturbed in certain surroundings, or only be happy in a specific natural setting. To share a message with these sensitive pets, you might need to sit outside or in their natural habitat with them, join in a nature-based activity, or intentionally "beam" a message into a natural object, such as a stone or bowl of water, to transfer it into

the pet. You can accomplish the last process using the exercise "Easy Stone Programming" in chapter 7. This exercise specifically shows how to transport energy through a stone. You can use the same process with any element, including water.

Remember, too, that a pet's feet or related body part are bud chakras and part of the tenth chakra. You can stroke or hold an environmentally sensitive pet's feet to sense their needs and send beneficial energy. My cat Johnny, after wandering outside, loved to have me hold his paws. Through them, I could sense the type of earth he had traveled upon—hills, muddy, dry, etc. Bud chakras are also found under the ear apparatus, so you can perform the same maneuver there.

Also pay attention to the secondary chakra found at the tip of a pet's tail or the equivalent. As you'll recall from chapter 3, this area attunes to what's occurring in the environment and also links to other dimensions. To sense the presence of other spirits, I used to watch the tip of Johnny's tail. For instance, the spirit of my deceased father would sometimes visit me. I knew he was there because Johnny's tail would suddenly start circling wildly. I could then hear my father's voice in my head, but I might not have listened if Johnny hadn't alerted me. Once, when a client entered the house, Johnny's tail performed the same circular dance. My client explained that she'd been hearing spirits lately. Johnny's tail had picked up on her invisible guides.

Physical Empathy: First chakra empaths relay information through their actions or inactions. They might shake, rattle, and roll, making their needs and challenges apparent through physical behaviors. A fish might swim near the side of the tank to flash an injured fin, or a horse might butt into you to insist on a ride. You might also experience psychic deliveries through bodily sensations that mirror what's occurring in your pet. A sudden ache in your fingertip might indicate that your bird's claw is damaged. A flash of pain registering in all your fingers and toes might clue you in to an impairment in your caterpillar. If your pet doesn't want to do something, they might plop down and refuse to budge, or send psychic sensations that will cause you to become lethargic.

Usually, a physically empathic pet will want you to communicate physically. Stroke or hold them. Give them what they need. Feed them. Clean their habitat. Psychically, you can formulate a physical sensation in your body and project it at the pet; the exercise in this chapter will show how to do this by sending healing streams. The key is to sense what you want the pet to feel in your own body.

Emotional Empathy: Second chakra empaths relate through emotions. They'll indicate what's up by expressing feelings or sending you the psychic impression of a feeling, which you'll feel in your body as if it's your own. When near your frog, you might suddenly feel sad—or happy, angry, or otherwise—because the frog is emotional. To instruct an emotional pet, express your feelings or use the exercise provided in this chapter to send a psychic impression.

Mental Empathy: These third chakra pets are thinkers, but you won't see a cartoon bubble with words above their heads. Rather, you'll receive intuitive hunches about their thoughts, beliefs, and judgments. You'll want to communicate to them through the gut sense in your solar plexus. You'll see what I mean during the exercise at the end of this chapter!

Spiritual Intuition

Overall, spiritual empaths communicate in high-level ways; frankly, these can be hard to recognize because the key mediums are awareness and consciousness. Having said that, here are clues for interacting through the five forms of spiritual intuition:

Relational Empathy: Relational pets relay their love-based and healing needs heart-to-heart. These pets will make your heart sing—or thump, sense, or emote—to share their relationship or healing needs. You'll feel prompted to respond if you love the pet. When generating a heart-based message for these loving pets, you'll want to concentrate on how much you love them. Even if delivering a verbal message, pay attention to the love in your heart. For instance, I once picked up a stray for my oldest son years ago. I drove to a farm to obtain it. I was greeted by a large man. I explained that I was picking up the stray.

"Which stray?" He asked. I felt confused. "The one from last week?" I asked, puzzled.

He looked at me and yelled, "Come here, G-d dammit!"

About forty dogs ran up to him. One was missing his hind legs. The farmer had invented a set of wheels that allowed him to run with only his front paws. My new dog appeared too. The moral? The dogs couldn't care less about their names. They responded to the farmer's big heart.

Spiritual Empathy: A spiritually empathic pet is motivated to teach or model spiritual principles, often indicating what is right or wrong for them or yourself. If they disapprove of what you're doing, they'll emanate a sense of wrongness. The opposite is also true; you might simply feel their approval. Typically, it's easiest to send a spiritual message to a pet if you use your visual skills, envision the communication in a white bubble, and send them the message. I'll show you how to accomplish this in this chapter's exercise.

Harmonic Empathy: When a pet's energy assures you that all is right with the world, you're receiving a ninth chakra message. For instance, my dog Honey frequently sits in the passenger seat of the car. When I make the correct turn, he acts content. When I make a wrong turn, he sends vibes that make me edgy. He does the same when I'm making a decision. I was once going to accept a date with a person I didn't know well. Honey was sitting near me. He made me feel disturbed. I decided not to go on the date. Later, I found out that this man wasn't who he appeared to be. In fact, he used a fake name.

If you want to relay a ninth chakra message to a pet, fill your diaphragm with your sense of harmony or disharmony in relation to a topic. Breathe that sense toward them. It's easiest to do this if you send the perception in a bubble of gold, a technique covered in this chapter's exercise.

Force Empathy: Do strange happenings occur in the environment when you're around your pet? Does your pet affect you supernaturally? A force-based pet can operate both ways. Perhaps they call a gale that prevents you from attending a party. Maybe you sense a force pushing you off a hiking path, only to avoid a galloping horse. To communicate with these types of pets, you need to employ a non-eleventh chakra gift such as moving your hands when directing them, imagining that wind or water are delivering your message to them, or asking that a spiritual force bring them the healing or information you want them to receive.

Verbal Intuition

A pet's verbal messages can be heard inside your head or through your ears. Via your physical ears, you might hear a song on the radio when thinking about your pet; the message fits perfectly. Pets can sometimes speak for themselves, too, via a meaningful message wrapped within their noises. For instance, my bunny rabbit would hiccup when hungry, so I'd feed it. It would burp a thank you. Of course, through your clairaudience, you might also hear your pet's verbal audition—a bark, song, splash, or whatever—inside your head. Your internal system will translate the pet's language into your own; a spiritual guide can do the same.

Sending a verbal message to a pet employs the same protocol as receiving one. Many pets know how to interpret our words, verbal cues, or tone of voice, which means that we need to be careful about what we say and how we say it. I run my dogs at a park every morning and they know all my verbal cues, including the phrase, "Let's go to the little section." We usually run in the bigger plot of the park and then move into the smaller one. However, I can also simply think the phrase "little section" and they will run to the correlated gate. Hence, if our pet is able to hear our thoughts, we can communicate through our clairaudience.

Visual Intuition

Many pets communicate through psychic pictures. Dreams especially can include images of or visitations from pets, alive or deceased, that convey information. Psychic visions might also flash into your mind, providing insight from your pet. Then again, some pets showcase their messages visually. They might point to or pick up something that's pictorially important. Lucky, my yellow Labrador, once scooped up a photograph of a friend. I called him, only to discover that *he* had been thinking of calling *me*.

One of the easiest ways to deliver a visual message to a pet is to formulate an image and psychically send it to your pet. You can also add a psychic image or a color to any other type of message, from verbal to empathic. I'll show you how to use your visual process in this chapter's exercise.

Mystical Intuition

Mystical pets can combine the four intuitive styles to form a collective ability. This means that the mystically intuitive pet has access to a universe of spirits. If we've known a pet in a past life, it's often relatively easy for them to use their mystical qualities to communicate with us. This is because a soul-to-soul contact opens all the intuitive gateways.

Recall that the shoulder blades, also called the brachial or key chakra, are linked to the eighth chakra. Through this area, pets and humans can convey information to each other. By holding or stroking this region, you can receive and send intuitive data, from sensations to images.

Energetic Clues for Communicating with Pets

If you'd like a few clues about selecting an intuitive style to use with your pet, in this section I'll outline the seven basic pet categories and indicate which of the general styles and specific chakras the beings in each category usually employ intuitively. I'll also provide a few other directives, but first I want to give two pieces of advice.

First and foremost, pay attention to your pet's unique energetic signature, which you figured out in chapter 2. You know your pet better than anyone else. If your pet seems highly verbal, use the verbal intuitive style. If your pet never sits still, go with first chakra physical intuition. Go with your gut or try different schematics and see what works.

Second, take a hint from any elements strongly connected to your pet. Fish swim in water. Water relates to the second chakra, as shown in the chakra descriptions in chapter 3. Try relating to your fish emotionally and see if that works. Stick a finger in the water so you can better sense what a fish is feeling. Birds fly in the air and are therefore extremely third chakra, so use mental empathy. The point is to merge the information in this book with your personal knowledge.

Shy of these bread crumbs, I've provided the following cheat sheet to help you figure out your pet's intuitive preference.

> **Mammals:** Mystical intuition. Can always use fourth chakra relational empathy or eighth chakra mystical empathy.
>
> **Rodents:** Physical intuition. Consider employing third chakra mental empathy, as rodents pay attention to details.
>
> **Birds:** Physical, spiritual, and verbal intuition. Within the physical intuition category, make sure you access third chakra mental empathy, which incorporates the air element. Consider unique particulars as well. For instance, pet ducks, geese, turkeys, and chickens dwell in flocks, meaning they are very second chakra, or emotionally intuitive, and maybe even fourth chakra, or relationally empathic. You'll also want to employ fifth chakra verbal intuition if your bird caws, quacks, croaks, or otherwise talks a lot.
>
> **Reptiles:** Physical intuition. Employ first chakra physical empathy with all reptiles, as this energy center relates to survival. Then consider which element the reptile interacts with. A frog, for instance, might live both in the water and on the earth. Look up any related chakras (second and tenth) and add them to your repetoire.
>
> **Arthropods:** Physical intuition. The emphasis will be on first chakra physical empathy, as arthropods spend a lot of time assuring personal survival, but you might also potentially work with third chakra mental empathy, as arthropods are very cunning. As well, most of these natural beings have multiple legs, so you'll want to employ tenth chakra environmental empathy. Usage of other chakras depends on the species. For instance, add second

chakra emotional empathy for water crabs. Know that spiders are particularly complicated. You might consider employing ninth chakra harmonic empathy as spiders teach balance; verbal intuition, in that spiders represent writing and communication; and even eleventh chakra force empathy because of their use of poison and webbing. If the arthropod has unusual or multiple eyes, you can also engage sixth chakra visual intuition.

Amphibians: Physical and spiritual intuition. Work with the chakra that relates to an amphibian's habitat, and also analyze their unique signature for their higher purpose to determine their spiritual chakra.

Aquatic Fish: Physical, spiritual, and visual intuition. Within the physical intuition venue, all fish relate through second chakra emotional empathy. Spiritually, many fish also access the seventh chakra, in that they represent higher wisdom. If the fish swims in a school, it might also employ its fourth chakra relational empathy. Also consider the species. Angelfish, which represent beauty, can engage through their sixth chakra visual intuition. They are also quite idealistic, so you can use ninth chakra harmonically empathic. Koi are a deeply mystical species and could be eighth chakra mystically empathic.

As a caveat, the more complicated the pet, the more options you have for communication, especially once you further analyze the nature of your pet based on its species and its particular energetic signature. For instance, mammals can access all chakras. A dog, which species is extremely loyal, also employs the heart (fourth chakra/relational empathy). An emotional therapy dog will also be highly attuned to an owner's emotions (second chakra/emotional empathy); is trained to respond to visual cues (sixth chakra/visual intuition); and serves a higher purpose (seventh chakra/spiritual empathy). If your pet is like my dog, Honey the Golden Retriever, it's quite verbal (fifth chakra/verbal intuition). And what if the dog's functions are more equivalent to those served by my guinea pig, Max, who ran the house when alive, and most likely, even now that he's dead? For certain, you'll have to access the pet's ability to command supernatural and natural forces (eleventh chakra/force empathy).

If the pet is truly complex, or you don't yet understand its nature, you can always relate through the fourth chakra/relational empathy. Simply greet the pet's messages with love and send your ideas back with love.

Another option is to consider the part of the limbic system that your pet represents. There are three main components of the human's neurological system. These are the limbic system, which governs survival instincts; the mammalian system, which enables bonding and closeness; and the consciousness system, which enables higher thinking. Chakras can be correlated to these three systems, a point hinted at in the section "It's All About Light and Sound" in chapter 3. There, I discussed the three main types of chakra groupings—physical, psychological, and spiritual. In general—for pets and people—chakras one and ten govern the limbic system and are physical; chakras two, three, and four rule the mammalian system and are psychological; and chakras five, six, seven, eight, nine, and eleven link to the consciousness system and are spiritual. Consider using the chakras that best suit the seven categories of pets, my next topic.

Limbic System: Reptiles are always limbic, as are very independent rodents, arthropods, and amphibians.

Mammalian System: Includes all mammals and birds, as well as members of the other five categories that live in packs.

Consciousness System: Includes many mammals and any dharmically evolved pet from the other categories. For instance, the caterpillar that knows it is already a butterfly is a highly conscious being.

One last clue: if you try and can't succeed, try, try again—but with a guide. Spiritual guides are great bridges for pet/human communication because they are able to relate to both pets and humans, since they aren't limited by form and language.

Every human being has at least two spiritual guides that serve them the entirety of their lives. It is the same with pets. Typically, one pet guide is ethereal in nature; perhaps it is an angel or another heavenly being. The other guide is usually a being that was once alive and is similar in form to the pet. For pets, this being might be a now-deceased member of their ancestry or species. It could also be a pet that they knew in this life who is now deceased. Not only are spiritual guides not limited by form, but they can convey a message in whatever language or intuitive style is required to pet or human.

To practice communicating with your pet and maybe connect with one of their spiritual guides, start with the following introduction to an important technique: Healing Streams of Grace.

Exercise
Using Healing Streams of Grace to Communicate with Your Pet

The Healing Streams of Grace exercise can be used with Spirit-to-Spirit to perform nearly any type of pet communication. In this book you'll also be taught how to use them to analyze problems, create solutions, send healing, and make smart pet decisions. The fundamental assumption that empowers this technique is recognizing that the Spirit generates endless waves of grace, with grace defined as love that empowers positive change.

The easiest way to picture the healing streams of grace—which I also call the streams, healing streams, or streams of grace—is as beams of sunlight. The sun is the Spirit and the sunbeams are the streams of grace, which are continually available to meet any need. When summoned, they will be delivered and remain attached until unnecessary. Once linked with a being's soul, mind, body, or subtle structure, these streams insert healing, education, or anything else that's required. You will employ them in this exercise to receive and send communiqués between you and your pet. Take a few breaths and undertake the following steps when you're ready:

> 1: **Prepare for Communication.** Gather writing instruments. You'll use the clues offered in this chapter to select a distinct chakra for the intuitive process. Start by considering your pet's category, species, personality, and energetic signature. Then write down which overarching style (physical, spiritual, verbal, visual, or mystical) you should tap into, which chakras within that category might be the most revealing, and any additional chakras and related gifts your pet reflects. Finally, choose a single chakra to operate through, and then

give thought to the chakra's elements. Know that it's best if your pet is present, but it doesn't need to be.

Subtle energies are empowered if you employ a physical representation of the chakric element while connecting with your pet. You can use water, a lit candle, a stone, or whichever tool makes sense. Then consider the most supportive environment to conduct this communiqué in. If your pet likes trees, sit outside. If your pet flies, open the windows (but don't let it escape)!

2: Perform Spirit-to-Spirit. Affirm your personal spirit, others' spirits, and, finally, the Spirit. Now focus on your pet.

3: Receive a Communiqué. Ask the Spirit to send healing streams into the chakra you're focusing on in your pet. These streams will pick up the pet's psychic message from that chakra and bring it into the same chakra within you. Remain still until you perceive the message. If you're confused, shift to your heart chakra and ask that the Spirit deliver the message there. And if nothing occurs, return to your notes about the pet's categorical style and select a different chakra within that grouping to use.

Now write down whatever comes to you. If your pet is highly visual, you can draw the message. Remain in this receptive state and ask questions aloud, in your head, or on paper while requesting that the Spirit bring you answers. If you still aren't receiving anything, ask the Spirit to select one of your pet's spiritual guides to bring you the message.

If your pet is present, you can also pay attention to how it's acting. Is it sending you a physical sign? Making sounds? Commanding forces to disturb you? Go with your gut to interpret these activities.

Sometimes a message is "delayed in the mail." You might receive a dream, sign, or other response at a later time. If nothing comes right now, assume you'll get a special delivery at a later time and move to the closing step in this exercise. Once you receive your pet's missive, you can return to this exercise and employ the next step, "Send a Communiqué." Otherwise, once you're clear about your pet's message, proceed to the next step.

4: *Send a Communiqué.* Once you have deciphered your pet's message or need, compose a response within your focus chakra. To do this, ask that the Spirit formulate a bubble made of healing streams within or in front of the chakra. Load the bubble with your message.

For instance, if you're employing your first chakra to send a message, feel the bodily sensation you want your pet to feel. Let the healing streams carry these sensations into the bubble. If you're composing a verbal message, speak that message psychically or aloud into the bubble. If you desire assistance, ask the pet's spiritual guide for assistance. That guide will bring your message into the bubble for you.

It can be quite useful to envision the bubble, even if you aren't officially employing the sixth chakra. It's always helpful to load an image or a color into the bubble before sending it to the pet. Create the image or pick the color depending on your pet's intuitive type. For instance, if you're sending a message to the pet's ninth chakra, fill the bubble with gold. If you want to stimulate a reaction in the pet's seventh chakra, use white.

Once the bubble is filled, ask the Spirit or the spiritual guide to deliver the bubble to your pet and to unpack it within their subtle system. Now pay attention to how your pet acts or intuitively responds. You can continue to communicate back and forth as long as you desire. Know that your pet might receive the message at a later time, so be patient. Whenever you sense your part of the process is done, move to the next step.

5: *Close.* With gratitude for this interaction, take a few deep breaths and return to your everyday state.

Thus equipped to communicate with your pet, you are ready to put everything together. Next, you'll learn ways to analyze a pet's issues by interpreting chakra-based and other subtle information.

Chapter Five

Energetic Issues: Conditions, Behaviors, and Diseases

No animal should ever jump up on
the dining room furniture unless
absolutely certain that he can hold
his own in the conversation.

Fran Lebowitz

There are peeves we all have with our pets. (As inferred by the quote beginning this chapter, in my house my pets really do insist on joining me at the dining room table!) A pet's behavior is only one of the many issues we must address to be responsible companions.

This chapter serves as the backbone for figuring out what might be causing pet problems from an energetic point of view. In later chapters you'll be performing more full-on analyses. To accomplish this goal, you'll require the data in this chapter.

First, I'll illustrate how behavioral, psychological, physical, and spiritual pet problems can originate in the subtle realms. Next, we'll revisit a point already made in this book, which is that subtle energies can transfer from place to place and being to being. This fundamental assumption will help you make sense of many subtle issues.

Then we'll dig in, reducing the nuts and bolts of a pet's problems to their most typical cause: trauma. Trauma is hard to treat through allopathic means. Viewing it through the lens of subtle energy is incredibly powerful, which is why we'll be focusing on trauma release through much of the rest of this book.

The next several topics will explore other causal issues, all examined through the subtle energy lens. Subjects include emotions, attachments, and microbes. Finally, I'll present an in-depth chart depicting a chakra-by-chakra analyses of pet problems, distinguished by physical, psychological, behavioral, and spiritual symptoms. I think you'll find this systematic approach to pet problems both fascinating and resourceful. You'll also benefit from the discussion about rescue animals presented after the analysis and by meeting a true-life rescue dog, Rover. We'll let Rover show us how all the data in this chapter can be integrated to care for the pets that have no place to call home.

All in all, you'll continually revisit this chapter. Today your pet might exhibit a specific need and tomorrow, another one. That's the nature of life. Members of the human and nonhuman nations are constantly changing.

The Energetic Origins of Your Pet's Difficulties

Meet four pet friends:

> **Parakeet:** Your parakeet's feathers are dusty and ratty, especially at the tips. What might be going on?
>
> **Ferret:** Ouch! Your pet ferret keeps biting you. You know that ferrets bite each other, but still…
>
> **Horse:** Your friend's horse rears when there are loud or disturbing noises. How should your friend better manage the horse? You have a secret suspicion. Your friend has always been scared of her own shadow. Could *she* be affecting her horse?
>
> **Dog:** Your dog keeps getting bacterial eye infections. You're tired of treating them with antibiotic drops. Is there a different way to solve the problem?

There are incalculable numbers of presenting challenges faced by your pets. Loosely, these can be systematized as behavioral, psychological, physical, and spiritual, but no matter the presentation of the problem, you'll stand a much better chance at relieving a problem by examining its underlying subtle energetic causes or factors.

I assisted the human companions of each of the four pets I just mentioned. What did I discover energetically?

Parakeet: The tips of a bird's wings are bud chakras, which are part of the tenth chakra. This energy center is complicated. It reflects the third stage of a pet's development, which involves the programming of karma and dharma into the genes and epigenes during conception. This chakra also attunes the pet to the surrounding environment.

In this case, a vet had already ruled out parasites and other testable diseases. The bird had also been put on a vitamin supplement, but to no avail. My client figured out that the bird's feathers went awry after a factory was erected in a nearby township. This meant that on the subtle (and maybe even physical) level, the bird was responding to the increased environmental toxins. After using Spirit-to-Spirit, I also saw that in an earlier life, this bird, then a parrot, had died when Europeans built processing plants in South America. In chapter 2 you learned that birds represent freedom, among other qualities. It seemed that the bird was responding to past-life karma triggered by this-life pollution, during which time the pollution was so strong that it lost its ability to fly—or be free. We used the pet communication methods you'll learn in chapter 6, along with the vibrational stone healing covered in chapter 7, and the condition cleared.

Ferret: Here we were dealing with the fifth chakra, which relates to communicating. The salient question was, what was Mr. Ferret communicating through the biting? It was easy to arrive at the answer. I had the client tune into the subtle energy conveyed through the biting. It was fun-loving. The ferret was playing! The human companion introduced different ways to merrily interact with the ferret and gave the ferret chewier foods. The biting stopped.

Horse: Psychologically, panic responses involve the first chakra, which relates to survival. The horse's owner knew that the breeder had yelled at the horse when it was young, so of course the horse was responding to early this-life trauma. The horse's human companion had also been mistreated when young. She too startled at loud sounds and agreed that the horse was probably also absorbing and mirroring her personal issues, in addition to acting out its own.

The horse's energetic signature underlined this assessment. Horses, as revealed in chapter 2, can be gun shy and oversensitive, but they also traverse the subtle planes of light and dark. The darkness within the horse's owner was easily relatable to the horse. Remember my brief introduction to attachments in chapter 1? I found an attachment called a cord between the horse and its owner. Through it, the horse kept taking on the owner's childhood terror and pain, overstimulating the already disturbed horse. In the end, the client and I worked to release the cord and clear the trauma in both parties, using processes you'll learn in this and the next few chapters. Gradually, both horse and human stopped overreacting.

Dog: Eyes relate to the sixth chakra, which governs physical but also psychic sight. As you'll learn in this chapter, bacteria store a being's repressed emotions. In this case, the dog started getting eye infections during middle maturity, the exact stage associated with the sixth chakra, during which time the predominant issues relate to self-image.

Dogs are loyal, above all, as you learned in chapter 2. The dog's eye infections had started when a child in the household was being bullied at school. Though the dog would curl up with the child at night, the bullying problem didn't go away. Based on its inability to serve the boy, the dog felt like a failure. The dog's resulting shame and grief was pocketed in the bacteria. In this case the child's parent needed to step up and help her child, which she did. I used the animal communication tools covered in chapter 5 to help the dog view itself as loving and loyal rather than a failure. In fact, I told it that its communication had brought the son's issue to the mother's attention. Over the next few weeks, the dog stopped getting eye infections.

How does energy so easily transmit from a single time period and being to another? Earlier we discussed the nature of the soul and other factors. The next section will fill in the rest of the energetic story.

Energetic Transference
How One's Energy Becomes Another's Energy

The fundamental key to subtle energy work is comprehending the ease with which subtle energy is transferred. This process applies to the transmission of all subtle energies, whether they are distinctively physical, psychological, or spiritual.

Recall our discussions of light and sound in chapters 1 and 3. That introductory material laid the groundwork for a further understanding of energetic transference. Healers, shamans, intuitives, philosophers, and even scientists have known across time that the physical form of a being is merely a step-down or step-up version of higher and faster or lower and slower vibrations of light and sound. Problems in these subtle energies become crystallized in the physical form. Chakras and other subtle structures are uniquely able to transmute one vibration of energy to another. Thus these energetic transformers create fields that oscillate in every direction away from the body central, even reaching other time-space continuums. As they reverberate, these fields interact with others' subtle fields as well as their biofields, which are the fields produced by bodily parts.

Through a being's subtle fields, energy is transferred from one being or object to another. As shared earlier in this book, a pet is more apt to take in external subtle energy if that energy resonates or matches the karmic or dharmic information in the soul, mind, or body. While energy exchanges can be lovely, serving to share love and healing, they can also create everything from a nuisance to a catastrophe. A pet can absorb energies underlying physical illnesses, emotional disruptions, dysfunctional beliefs, and more. It can lose vital energy in an attempt to support another pet or human companion. Energy can also be forced into a pet through trauma, the subject of the next section. That energy is quite hard for a pet to process and often causes serious damage. Because we can interact in subtle ways with a pet, as well as through physical actions and mediums, we can help free them from unhealthy energies and activate healthy energies. That is the basis of both healing and manifesting—healing being the release of unhelpful or harmful energies, and manifesting defined as the receiving of beneficial or supportive energies.

There are many tools that can help us perform these maneuvers for our pets. Basically, quantum physics suggests that the internal self shapes physical reality through mental and emotional projections. These projections affect the invisible fields outside of the self. We use this same principle to help our pets, sending energy through tools like intention, the conscious ability to set a direction; focus, the ability to decide an outcome; and prayer, the request for help from spiritual beings. We can also produce energetic change through the use of vibrational medicines, which shift the subtle energies in order to create physical impact.

Before we can shift energies from negative to positive, which we'll learn how to do in subsequent chapters, we must know what is wrong. We must search for the fundamental cause of all problems: trauma.

Causes of Pets' Problems

It's All About Trauma

Trauma underlies all pet problems, as well as pet/human challenges. In this section we'll examine the nature of trauma and the real issue creating it, which is subtle energetic forces. We'll also examine the challenges to clearing trauma.

What Is Trauma?

The most common definition of trauma is "a deeply disturbing event or experience." Of course, not all traumas are equally catastrophic; a pet might consider itself traumatized several times a day. My dogs love to insinuate that I'm traumatizing them when I'm eating steak, unless I share, which I usually do. When growing up, we had a bird named Peppy, who could open his cage and fly around the house at will. When my grandmother visited, we had to lock the bird cage; my grandmother was afraid of birds. Peppy was furious. Traumatized at some level, he would punish us for days by spreading bird scat around the house once he was let out. Then he would return to normal.

Trauma becomes a problem when the results of it are seemingly inescapable or irrevocable. This occurs when the effects can't be cleared because of the severity or chronic nature of the wounding or because of personal vulnerability. A severe trauma might occur when a pet is hit by a car and the vertebrae snaps. There is little chance the pet will fully recover. A chronic condition is exemplified by a pet that is left alone so frequently, it becomes depressed. What storyline might illustrate the effects of a personal vulnerability? Imagine that your pet already has an injured leg and is then lightly punched. That slight jolt might be all that's needed to cause a permanent limp.

Trauma can affect the smallest of creatures. When I was a child, I collected caterpillars and frogs. I would keep them in ornate boxes and aquariums for a few weeks and then let them go. One night I forgot to remove the boxes from my bedroom when my grandmother visited and slept in my room. She awoke to a room of caterpillars and frogs and screamed. Loudly. For a long time. Though I returned my pets to their safe havens, every one of them died within a day or two. They couldn't recover from the traumatizing situation.

Yes, even negative sounds can cause trauma. In fact, causes of trauma include the experience or witness of physical, sexual, emotional, and verbal abuse, or any combination of these factors, as well as neglect. Trauma also arises from intermittent abuse, which occurs when positive and negative events continually recycle, such as occurs when a pet is treated kindly when a human companion is sober and is battered when the companion is drunk.

When a trauma results in acute or long-term problems, the result is called post-traumatic stress disorder, or PTSD. In a pet, PTSD symptoms might be exhibited through behavior, psychological problems, physical illnesses or maladies, or even spiritual sensitivities, such as over- or under-psychism, or a mix of these issues. For instance, a pet given up for adoption will probably exhibit symptoms from each of these categories for a while with its new owner. It might jump up, act needy, be constantly ill, or take on the new human companion's feelings; the latter could occur if the pet is unconsciously attempting to "earn" its place. While typical treatments can help, including veterinarian care and good food, a physical analysis and set of solutions might be insufficient. To make a real difference, especially if everyday solutions aren't working, it's vital to unlock a situation at a subtle level, which requires understanding the subtle dynamics of trauma.

Basically, a pet can incur subtle energy damage and injury through two scenarios. The first happens if the incoming energies don't match the energetic signature of the pet. The second instigates if the causal energies match the signature too well.

When mismatched subtle frequencies are introduced into a pet's system, the incompatible energies create disorder and imbalance. Picture the pet that is naturally calm and easygoing. Now plop that pet in a daycare of toddlers. The bouncing energies will inevitably pass into the pet's subtle anatomy and eventually make their way into the physical system, causing the pet to feel and act rattled and overwhelmed.

Key to understanding the negative effects of others' energies is acknowledging that a living being cannot process energy that isn't its own. Mismatched energies are simply not recognized by physical or subtle systems, and so they cannot be easily dealt with or incorporated into the body. This statement applies to all sorts of subtle energies, including others' emotions. Energies that enter as psychic might remain psychic and transformed into challenges such as problematic thoughts, out-of-control feelings, or spiritual negativity, but they can also turn into physical challenges, including illnesses, aches and pains, and behavioral anomalies.

Of course, disruptive subtle energies might also match a pet's karma, familial patterns, or some other source of programming. Imagine that your cat was starved to death by an owner in a previous life. This trauma, carried forward in its soul, might cause your cat to hiss every time it sees its current cat sitter. You'll only understand the cat's reaction after uncovering the catastrophic past life.

Maybe the cat sitter was the long-ago owner. Or perhaps the cat triggers because the contemporary cat sitter only gives it minimal food when you're traveling. Either way, the situation stirs the echo of starvation. Subtle energies make their way into physical reality and the symptoms appear in a noticeable way.

If a disturbance is short-term or minuscule, the subtle system hardly blinks. Rather, it absorbs the difficulty and adapts. The irritant might or might not make it to the physical anatomy. Subtle damage only locks into the physical anatomy if the traumatizing subtle energies can't be cleared or assimilated.

How do negative subtle energies become locked into a pet in the first place? The answer is forces.

How Forces Create Trauma

A force is a wave or moving field that holds charged energies. When the charged energies carried in by a moving field are harmful, they create troublesome trauma. There are dozens of forces that can wound or traumatize and that can carry subtle energies that don't match those in a pet or that stir a pet's programming. But the basic idea behind harmful forces is that they transport negative subtle energies that leave subtle congestion and injuries.

Of course, a physical force can hurt a pet and leave a permanent blotch; we've established this fact. Physical recovery will be slower, if not impossible, if that physical force also contains subtle or negatively charged energies that are detrimental to that particular pet.

As understood through the commonplace view of trauma, a traumatic force might or might not be directly aimed at a pet. Damage incurs even if a pet is only in the vicinity of a negative force. There are several types of forces that can potentially carry destructive subtle energies; a short list follows:

- A natural force created by environmental
  elements such as fire or water.

- A physical force, which is a field that produces a physical effect.

- An emotional force, which is composed of feelings,
  thoughts, or a blending of the two.

- A verbal force, which contains thoughts or an audible message.

- A spiritual force, which contains energies from an entity (a
  disembodied soul), communications brought in from past lives,
  and data held in the epigenetic material from ancestors.

- An empty force, which is a field that doesn't contain the charges
  that a pet knows it should have. Think of the puppy's mom that
  doesn't love her puppy but nonetheless nurses it. Because the milk
  doesn't contain the subtle energy of unconditional love that the
  puppy unconsciously knows it should have, the puppy can end up
  feeling unlovable. No matter how much milk—or food or water—
  that puppy might take in as it grows, it might never feel satiated.

Bottom line: unless the negative (or empty) energies carried on the force are cleared or replaced with healthy charges, the energies (or conclusions about the missing energies) remain stuck in the pet. These issues can be transferred from one lifetime to another, causing continual disturbance, until the trauma is cleared.

It's not always easy to clear subtle charges. In fact, there are four factors that can make it difficult. First is the fact that these energies are invisible, although the resulting symptoms might not be. This makes it hard to pinpoint them. Imagine that your pet salamander was screamed at by a handler and told that it was a filthy creature. The handler's verbally nasty energies are now lodged in your salamander. Unless you use subtle energy tools, you'll have no idea why your salamander shies away from you.

The second complication is the fact that a pet will have its own reaction to a traumatizing force. Imagine that a turtle was mishandled by an angry child. The anger is now locked in your turtle, which might bite as an attempt to work out the feelings.

A third hurdle is explained by the nature of energetic transference. A force forms a pathway. When a force drives into a pet, it creates an entrance wound. If the force moves straight through the system, it also forms an exit wound as well as a pathway in between these points. Typically, the exit wound is right across from the entrance wound. For instance, if an upset child pinches a gerbil on its arm, the physical force, which also carries the child's hurt and pain, will probably exit through the opposing shoulder, depositing subtle feelings along the way. If there is a block in the system, however, the force can vector off, perhaps exiting through the gerbil's hip or shoulder.

These internal blocks might be primarily physical, created by inflammation or a cyst; emotional, composed of stored or repressed emotions; mental, consisting of false beliefs or untrue perceptions; or spiritual, formed of karmic programs or others' psychic energies. Sometimes the already-present congestion is so compact that the traumatizing force is completely impeded and becomes wedged near the block. This stuck area can eventually turn into just about anything, including a tumor, psychological imbalance, or extreme behavior.

As stated, a force can penetrate the body but also an auric field, soul, mind, or a chakra. No matter what, the echo of the force is recorded in the chakra that matches the incoming frequencies. For instance, if the damaging force carries a survival threat, the energies of that force will lodge in the first chakra, which governs security. If a pet is yelled at, the verbal force will be remembered by the fifth chakra, which relates to communication. Injuries will be reflected in the matching chakra and its correlated field no matter where the force enters, exits, or gets stuck. The only exception, as introduced in chapter 1, occurs if a force penetrates an auric field but isn't severe enough to land immediately in the chakra. Sooner or later, however, it will be deposited, unless it's cleared first. Toward that end, I recommend you use the technique featured in chapter 7, "Additional Tip: The Acupoint for Releasing Shock," to clear a trauma right after it's occurred.

A force is most damaging if incurred during a chakra's developmental stage. If this happens, the chakra will shape around the negativity. For instance, if a pet is told it's revolting while in the sixth stage—and sixth chakra time period—of development, it has an increased chance of developing a physical malady that will make it look dreadful or a bacterial infection that might cause eyesight issues.

The fourth obstacle to clearing a pet's trauma is that under severe stress, the physical and subtle bodily systems send the self into shock. In the body, the thalamus, a part of the brain, along with other mechanisms, blocks the self from emotionally processing the ordeal. We can't let feelings or physical pain get in the way of reacting to a challenge! Once the stress is over, the body is designed to release the inner self from the shock, allowing the pet's feelings to catch up so the pet can adapt to the fallout. The subsequent discharge of emotional, mental, and other energies should then clear the forces, inviting recovery.

Shock is biomechanical, but it's also subtle. After a traumatic incident, the chakras, especially the chakra most affected by the trauma, form a bubble of subtle energy around the injured or traumatized self, freezing it in time and space. The rest of the self can now (hopefully) apprise the situation and deal with it. Over time, the traumatized self can deal with its reactions and exit the bubble. When the traumatic forces are too strong, overwhelming, or consistent, or the other aspects of the self can't deal with the problem, neither can the traumatized self. So there remains the wounded self, imprisoned within its initial impressions of the calamitous event.

Energy attracts energy. The traumatized self in the subtle bubble now has a karmic issue. It will attract situations similar to what put it in the bubble as an unconscious way to free itself. The trauma will repeat again and again until the self is released from the subtle shock.

All traumatized selves contained in shock bubbles are transferred into the soul at death and are delivered karmically into the new body during preconception and conception, specifically into the related chakras' outer wheels. Thus might a pet unconsciously draw similar traumas to it during the next life, hoping that at some point, the shocked selves will dismantle the bubble and come out to play.

There is a trick to releasing subtle energy trauma. Since traumatic energies are conveyed from outside to inside, they are best released the same way. An external helper is needed—like you! In order to fully assist your pet with releasing trauma, however, it's vital to have a better understanding of emotions, one of the chief energies that get stuck in a pet, but also one of the energies that can make it all better.

Emotions
Of Havoc and Healing

Emotions underlie many pet challenges, especially if they trigger karma. As well, subtle emotions carried on forces frequently encourage the formation of subtle shock bubbles and cause problematic internal reactions. You'll be best able to assist your pet by using processes such as those covered in chapter 6. But first, you have to differentiate between feelings, beliefs, and emotions.

Simplistically, feelings are produced in the enteric nervous system and serve as messengers for the body. Beliefs are mainly created by the brain and central nervous system. Emotions are formulated by feelings and beliefs. Let's take a look at these three energies, both physically and subtly, as they pertain to humans but also to pets. A pet's emotional process is quite similar to a human's.

In the body, feelings are largely generated within the enteric nervous system, also called the "second" or "gut" brain of the body. In a person, this nervous system is actually a sheath of about 100 million nerves that are embedded in the gastrointestinal system. These nerves work together to manage digestion but also moods and feelings. In fact, moods and digestive processes are quite interdependent. For example, the feelings generated by the enteric nerves are affected by digestion, which is influenced by the trillions of bacteria found in that bodily area. In humans, the enteric cauldron also operates like a petri dish that brews the conditions for problems including osteoporosis and autism.

The enteric system operates independently of the brain but also communicates with it. In fact, about 90 percent of the fibers in the vagus nerve, the chief connection between the brain and other parts of the body, send information from the gut to the head brain, not the other way around (Hadhazy 2010). Based on this fact, scientists have figured out that microbes flow upward from the enteric to the head brain along the vagus nerve, establishing the conditions for diseases including Parkinson's and Alzheimer's, along with mental imbalances, depression, and anxiety (Sanders 2016, Main 2017).

Feelings are not dangerous or bad. In fact, every chakra hosts its own set of feelings that enables that chakra to respond to internal needs and the external environment. You see, on the subtle level, every feeling provides a message that, if respected, leads to a positive outcome. Following is a rendering of the five basic feelings, their meanings, and what we can achieve if we respect a feeling in our pets.

CHART: *Feelings and Their Meanings*

Feeling	Meaning	Achievement
Fear	There is danger; must change course	Safety
Sadness	The form of love has shifted; must search for a different form of love	Bonding
Anger	Boundaries are insufficient; must establish different ones	Empowerment
Disgust	Something or someone is toxic	Riddance and avoidance of toxicity
Joy	More of the same is desired	More joy

The brain also produces feelings, but mainly in reaction to conclusions about life events. Most of the brain-based beliefs are responses from the limbic system to survival threats. This system, which includes the amygdala, determines which of the four Fs we might select to respond to stress. These reactions are fight, flight, freeze, and fawn. Fight encourages the establishment of boundaries for self-protection, flight leads to disengagement and buys time to find safety, freeze recognizes that resistance is futile, and the fawn response invites compromise and negotiation (Walker, n.d.). Trauma-induced beliefs will affect the chemicals that actually cause feelings, including neurotransmitters, chemicals, and hormones. These feelings are mainly shaped by the beliefs held by the brain in regard to a being's experiences. We have countless beliefs, but they all reduce to two simple categories: "I am separate" and "I am connected." We discussed the vital differences between these two core beliefs in chapter 2.

Feelings (enteric nervous system) and beliefs (the brain) can operate somewhat separately from each other, but the power of both is multiplied when feelings and beliefs conjoin to form emotions. An emotion occurs when one or more feelings and beliefs are merged.

Emotions are not bad. They motivate. They compel movement. Emotions are only problematic when a feeling becomes permanently bonded with a separation-based belief. For instance, imagine that during the third chakra stage of development, which involves learning about personal power and structure, a human yells at a puppy that is peeing in the house. "You are dumb and worthless," the human screams, directing a traumatic force at the puppy. The puppy feels shame and fear and arrives at an internal conclusion that it's too stupid to be trained. Ever after, the puppy will get scared and embarrassed when it has to pee and won't believe it can hold the urine until getting outside—so it won't.

As you can surmise, we have to dismantle emotions to assist our pets and free them from the bondage of destructive emotions. You'll learn how to do this in chapter 6.

There is another type of binding to be aware of. It is an energetic attachment. I've alluded to subtle attachments several times already; it's time to discuss them more fully.

Energetic Attachments
The Connections That Harm

We've established the role of trauma in creating disastrous challenges for our pets, and we know that a pet attracts the same types of trauma—and even the same beings or types of beings—that caused the trauma, until the subtle energies are untied. One of the mechanisms that initiates and reinforces trauma, but also causes re-traumatization, are subtle energetic attachments, also called bindings.

Attachments are subtle energy bonds that affix into the soul, mind, chakra, auric field, or bodily part. They also can be anchored in the epigenetic material or just about anything else. There are two basic types of attachments. The first are cords. These operate like electrical wires through which energy flows, acting like a contract that determines who gets or loses. The easiest way to describe the energies exchanged is in relation to the chakras.

No matter where a cord is anchored in a being's system, it is also fastened into the related chakra. The energy can either flow one way, from at least one contract holder to another, or two ways, in which an actual exchange occurs. For example, imagine that a cord exists between your pet and you, secured into your pet's first chakra and your second chakra. How might a one-way flow work? Maybe you're feeling really sad and the cord transfers life energy from your pet into you to provide assistance, leaving your pet exhausted. In a two-way exchange, your emotions might also pass into the pet, even while their life energy is sent to you. In return, your pet might become both exhausted and emotionally unstable.

As in this example, the pet is usually at the energetic disadvantage in a pet/human relationship. As revealed by their energetic signatures, pets are usually service oriented. Most frequently, they lend their healthy energy to a beloved human and absorb the human's undealt-with emotions, difficult issues, and even diseases. (We'll look at the energies involved in energetic microbial transfers in the next section.) When this happens, the pet will express what they've taken on, even to the point of serious illness. At this point, the limiting side of their species' signature activates. Limitations are described in page 38's section "Species Codes: All the Many Offerings" in chapter 2. The human might now become quite frustrated with the pet, even though the pet is simply mirroring the human's issue. Of course, sometimes the opposite occurs. As your pet's human, you might take on your pet's challenges and offer them supportive energy. When this happens, you'll be unable to figure out what's wrong with you—and why your pet might seem so happy about it.

Cords can link a pet to a person or another being but also to invisible forces and entities. An entity is a disembodied soul. Forces are powerful entities that no longer hold a form of any sort. I add the term "dark" to words like entity, soul, or force to describe their nature, which is stealthy, cruel, and manipulative. Adding the word "dark" also helps me differentiate traumatic forces from conscious forces. Because a dark force or entity hampers a pet's growth and health, another term I use for these energies is "interference."

No matter the label, remember that there are at least two attachment sites involved in a cord. As explained in relation to cords already, the type of energy being exchanged is determined by the lock-in sites. Imagine that a cord exists between a pet and a dark entity and that the cord attaches to the pet's seventh chakra and the dark entity's second chakra. The exchange might involve a dumping of the entity's undesirable emotions into the pet's brain and a leeching of the pet's spiritual light by the entity's emotional self. In the end, your pet might appear overemotional and unaware of the effects of its actions on others.

A pet can be connected to an interfering being but so can a pet and its human. Depending on their energetic signature, a pet might think it should battle the human's interference. While playing white knight, it becomes hurt in the process.

For example, I once worked with a hamster who had a huge tumor under its armpit. If you review page 89's chart, "A Pet's Twenty-One Secondary Chakras," you'll discover that armpits are a secondary chakra representing acceptance by the clan. Just before the tumor grew, the hamster's human had been excommunicated by the Catholic Church. Attached to the human was the dark entity that had engineered this shaming event. The hamster had corded into the human-entity attachment in attempt to rescue its human clan member, who was, ironically, dealing with a church clan issue. We released all three co-participants in the binding through processes you'll learn in chapter 6. Within a few weeks the tumor shrunk significantly, and what was left was determined to be benign.

There is another type of attachment. I call them "holds." They operate like implants that restrict the victim. Some holds tell others how to mistreat the victim. Yet other holds limit a victim's prosperity, appetite, or emotional expression. The effect on the pet depends on which chakra anchors the hold, which is consciously or unconsciously placed on a pet by an external being or force.

What are some of the attachments or negative energetic influences that might influence your pet? Following is a brief synopsis of these two types of attachments, as well as a discussion about responsibility. It's easy to feel guilty or overly responsible for a pet's problem or even their death if an attachment to you is involved. It's important to understand the reality of personal responsibility and role of the soul in the existence of attachments. This knowledge will help you assist your pet and also stop you from blaming yourself for their issues.

Cords

The Attachments That Bind

Cords are attachments that operate between contract holders. The two types of cords and ways to recognize their existence are as follows:

> **Common Cords:** The common cord is an energetic tubule that looks like a garden hose linking two or more beings. There is a one-way or two-way exchange of energy through the cord. The exchange is often imbalanced, usually involving the introjection of toxic energy and the loss of healthy energy in one party and the loss of unhealthy energy and the gain of healthy energy in the other.

> **Life Energy Cords:** These special cords always involve the forfeiture of life energy, or first chakra energy, from one of the contract holders. This might be a one-way cord in which that's the basic exchange, but a two-way exchange might also occur, with negative energies being deposited in the party losing the life energy.

Symptoms of Cords

How do you know if a pet has a cord and which type might be involved? I'll describe the symptoms indicating cords that are pet-pet, pet-person, and pet-entity and help you differentiate between a common and life energy cord.

Typically, with a pet-to-pet common cord, the pets will be highly needy toward each other but oppositional. If one pet is calm, the other will be restless. If one is well, the other will be sick. In the case of a life energy cord, only one pet will benefit from the relationship. The pet stealing the energy will be healthier, happier, and more lovable than the other.

If a common cord exists between a pet and a person, the same symptoms that occur pet-to-pet can appear. The pet might gain energy when the human loses it, and so on.

If a life energy cord exists pet-to-person, there is always a loss of life energy from one contract holder and the appearance of that energy in another. Usually it is the pet that will appear exhausted, ill, or fatigued. However, as with a common cord, energies can also be deposited in the party losing the life energy. In the example just given, the tired pet might also reflect the energy being dropped in.

If either type of cord exists between you and your pet, you'll sense a physical tightness in the bodily- or chakra-based area that holds your side of the cord. If it's located in your auric field, you'll feel a tug in that space around the body. And if your pet is corded to an entity, the pet will sometimes stare into space, react to "nothing," have disturbing dreams, or constantly bite, pick, or itch at a bodily area that doesn't appear problematic.

Holds

The Attachments That Limit

There are various types of holds. I'll describe each and show how to pinpoint their existence.

> Curses: These attachments are constructed from multiple strands of energy and psychically look like a mess of pasta noodles. Curses are cast on a being or group and hold the victims in bondage, operating much like a spell.
>
> If a pet is afflicted with a curse, it will be extremely unfortunate in the life area related to the affected chakra and auric field. The pet might constantly attract abusive people, other pets that misbehave around them, or an array of afflictions and illnesses. For instance, I once worked with a client who had an ant farm. One ant was always stuck in the corners. For the heck of it, I asked the Spirit, using Spirit-to-Spirit, to release the ant from any curses. I assumed the ant rejoined the colony as it never appeared

in the corner again. I don't know exactly how a curse was cast on an ant, but still!

Marker: These energetic contracts psychically look like an X and are engraved over an auric layer, chakra, or body part. They operate like a curse that tells others how to treat the affected.

Symptoms of a marker include recurring problems that can be tracked to a chakra. If the pet is constantly getting into scary scrapes, there might be an X on the first chakra. If other pets or people continually get angry with the pet, there could be an energy marker on the second chakra, and so on.

Possession: Through possession, an entity takes control of all or part of a pet, including the body. The hold will psychically appear like a handle that the entity can lift, or a veil that can be parted, so it can penetrate the pet.

When an influencing entity takes over, the pet might act strangely out of character. It might shake, as if trying to get free. You might also sense or see a being enter and exit your pet's eyes, giving you the chills. Or perhaps, a part of the pet's body might seem to operate in a disjointed way. As an example, I once worked with a dog that was corded to its former owner, who had recently died. That owner had been a mean and abusive older man. Whenever the dog was around the dead man's son, whom the owner had hated, the dog would become enraged and its mouth would jerk. I sensed that the dog was possessed by the dead man. We cleared the hold, using techniques from chapter 6, and the dog forever returned to its meek and mild self.

Deflection: Deflection occurs when an attachment that looks like a mirror covers the entirety or a part of an auric field. It functions like an armor that rejects whatever positive energy could be attracted to the related chakra. For instance, if the deflecting film lies over the heart, the pet will rebuff love. If it's over the bud or tenth chakra, the pet might be allergic to nearly everything in the environment.

Attachments and Responsibility
The Ethics Behind a Binding

As explored, attachments can exist between—or be created by—any and all types of beings. Their consequences range from mild to devastating; because of this, we want to assist our pet with releasing attachments affecting them.

It's not uncommon to discover that we are one of the participants in a pet attachment. This finding can make us feel horribly guilty, especially if the consequences of an attachment are severely acute or highly negative. Conversely, we might also learn that an attachment between a pet and the self is causing a disruption in our own life. That can make us feel angry. How do we deal with the variety of reactions that arise within us if we're involved in a pet attachment?

I constantly assist my human clients with what is ultimately a question of responsibility in relation to attachments and issues in general. Simplistically, I say this: *We are not responsible for another's issues, which includes the reasons that a pet might unconsciously hold on to an attachment to us.*

On the other side of the coin is an additional truth: While we aren't responsible for another's issues, we *are* responsible for our own issues and our responses to another's issues. This means that we do need to act self-responsibly and with integrity if we're involved in an attachment with our pet. By cleaning up our side of the street—and going a step further by helping our pet address their issues—we can fulfill our karmic and dharmic commitments. Moreover, we can also uphold the contract between the human and nonhuman nations discussed in chapter 1.

In no way am I saying that we—or our pet—is responsible for the *cause* of traumas that are induced by others. Even if our pet carries a karmic issue into this life, that pet isn't responsible for being beaten, neglected, or otherwise mistreated during this life. Same for you. Realistically, major issues, such as those that are created or held in place by attachments, are very hard to heal alone. That's one of the reasons that humans and pets have spiritual guides, which stand ready to assist on every level. This is also one of the reasons that your pet might need your help in uncovering and resolving challenges, even if an attachment between the two of you is instigating some of the pet's problems. We really can be a source of love and healing for our pets, and if a pet/human attachment is harming us, we can turn to the Spirit, our spiritual guides, and other people for assistance.

In relation to attachments, I generally find that the key to recovery starts with uncovering the unconscious reason or cause for an attachment. This knowledge provides the undercurrent needed to shift the energetics holding an attachment in place for the self or a pet.

Consider the pet that is corded to you via its first chakra. Through this cord, it is absorbing your physical illness and sending you its own life energy. Consequently, your pet is physically ill and constantly fatigued. Upon discovering that you're the source of the attachment, you might feel really guilty. You are causing your pet to be sick and tired! The truth is that your pet's soul is unconsciously motivated to own this cord, so it has a reason to engage in the energetic contract establishing the cord. This means that you aren't responsible for the pet's participation in the cord, although you can assist the pet in rethinking its unconscious decision so it can then decide to release the cord. Implicit is the need to excavate yourself to discover the reasons why you are participating in this cord as well.

There are two main reasons that beings, including pets, people, and entities, establish attachments. The first is love. Our souls long to assist each other, even to the point of causing ourselves harm. The second is survival. If the unconscious self perceives that the only way to survive or meet its vital needs is to agree to an exchange of energy, it will share in an attachment, even to the point of harming the self or another. The latter rationale might very well be a reaction to being manipulated, so it's important to help the survival-motivated contract holder discover a healthier way to become safe.

The key to releasing all attachments is forgiveness. If our involvement in an attachment has been harming our pet, we must forgive ourselves. We do this by figuring out if our inner or soul-based motivation was love or survival-based, or both. Our self-awareness allows us to find a different way to bond with our pet. We can also use the tools provided in this book, such as pet communication, to help a pet discover its reasons for participating in an attachment so it, too, can forge a truly healthy connection, like the simple giving and receiving of love. If we're being harmed because of energy we're taking in from—or losing to—a pet, we must forgive ourselves for the unconscious reasons we attached to our

127

pet. All participants in an attachment have something to gain from forgiving themselves and the others involved for having participated in the binding.

We'll be dealing with how to heal attachment concerns in following chapters. But first, let's take a look at the energetics of microbes, one of the other major issues affecting all pets.

The Subtle Energies in Microbes

What Really Makes Your Pet Sick—and Why

Microbes are physical but also subtle organisms. Because subtle energies underlie physical energies, we could make the case that your pet doesn't "catch" a microbe; rather, it first "catches" the subtle energetic conditions related to the microbe. The actual infection follows. Because of this, it's vital to understand the subtle energetics of the most plaguing pet microbes.

Microbes are living beings. Because of this, each brand has its own energetic signature. A microbe's signature causes it to interface with a host in specific ways, always at a cost to the host. However, the host is part of that transaction. By helping your pet clear the reasons it's vulnerable to a particular microbe, you can help it release that microbe.

My own work has determined the following microbes relate to a pet in the stated ways:

Bacteria

Bacteria store a pet's repressed or unfelt feelings. Usually these are feelings that the pet doesn't want to feel or are feelings stuck in the traumatized self, which, as you remember, are trapped in a shock bubble. I once helped one of my dogs clear a bacterial infection when he was young by assisting him with expressing a plethora of "negative" feelings.

My adoption of my current Honey the golden retriever included flying him in from the breeder to our home. When I picked him up at the airport, he was barking incessantly. Honey was obviously traumatized from the two days in airports and planes. He immediately developed a bacterial infection. I used the communication devices covered in chapter 5 to invite him to release his feelings, and the infection went away.

Parasites

Parasites feed off a pet's physical and subtle energy. Not only do parasites steal the healthy physical energy of a pet, such as nutrients and fluids, but they also steal positive subtle energies, such as happy feelings and subtle elements. When alive, they also discharge their waste, and when dying give off toxic gas, thus further poisoning their host.

When a pet gets a parasite, it's because something or someone is already feeding off the pet. This might be another pet, an entity, or a human. An attachment is often involved. Healing involves searching for the cords that keep the pet or a part of the pet in this draining pattern; you'll learn how to release cords in chapter 6.

Different parasites operate in differing ways:

> Protozoa: These single-cell organisms can only live within—and multiply in—a host. Basically, they distribute the negative energies of the external parasite (person, other pet, entity) throughout the host's body. This means that you must clear the parasitic energy through all chakras, not only one.

> Helmiths: These worm parasites, including flatworms and pinworms, affect the attacked bodily and chakra area. For instance, intestinal worms feed off a host's emotions and leave behind their own undesirable emotions. Therefore, these type of worms are second chakra in nature.

> Ectoparasites: These parasites live on the host and steal energy from the related auric field. For instance, skin-based organisms feed off the first auric field. Ectoparasites that live in the hair—or wings, gills, or related body part—are affecting the tenth chakra.

Yeast, Fungi, and Molds

At one level, yeast, fungi, and molds are similar to parasites. They steal energy and deposit waste. The main difference is that these organisms also hold others' emotions. For instance, candida, when appearing in the intestines, relates to the second chakra. The candida organisms live off the physical nutrients but also emotions that the pet has absorbed from living beings outside of it. Releasing the candida will therefore require sending the absorbed emotions back to their original owner. Release the feelings and you'll help release the yeast, fungus, or mold.

Viruses

A virus is a microorganism that reproduces in the body at an astonishing rate. Viruses can infect any natural being and even overtake bacteria. Technically, viruses can't reproduce without a host, making them parasites.

To understand a virus, read through the description of parasites. To this information, add an additional qualifier. Quite typically, viruses are corded to a "mother brain" outside the body. This governing force might be an entity, group of entities, human companion, or even a "miasm," a matrix of programs that hold the memories and programs of a pet's ancestors, thus serving as familial karma. If you release the viruses from the cord, the body can better slough off the infection.

You'll learn subtle energy techniques to help work with the microbial material in following chapters. Most of the healing work will also require performing a chakra-by-chakra analysis, however, which is why I'm providing the next section. And then, in order to give you a great example of how to put together all the information presented in this chapter, I'm going to follow the analysis with a feature on a rescue dog. When we adopt these very special canines—in fact, when we rescue *any* pet from a shelter or a challenging situation—we face immense problems, but we're also presented the opportunity to save a life and earn a friend. To give one of these pets a place to call home is to stretch the walls of our hearts that much more.

Chakra	Color	Trait	Pet Type
1	red	physical, survivalistic	reptiles
2	orange	emotional, creative	aquatics
3	yellow	mental, structural	birds
4	green	relating, healing	amphibians
5	blue	communicative, clairaudient	arthropods
6	violet	visual, clairvoyant	rodents
7	white	spiritual, conscious	mammals

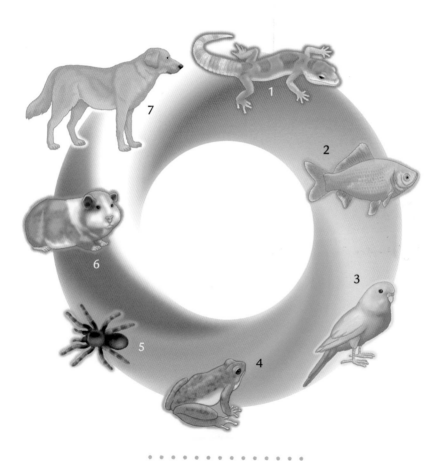

• • • • • • • • • • • • • •

The Energy of Our Companion Pets

Each of the seven types of pets discussed in this book bonds with us
in unique ways. This image reveals the most fundamental differences
between types in relation to the seven in-body chakras.

Chakra	Color	Purpose
1	red	survival, security
2	orange	emotions, creativity
3	yellow	mentality, structure
4	green	relating, healing
5	blue	communicating, clairaudience
6	violet	vision, clairvoyance
7	white	spirituality, consciousness
8	black or silver	mysticism
9	gold	higher purpose, harmonizing
10	brown	grounding, earth connections
11	pink	supernatural and natural forces
12	clear	unique to each purpose

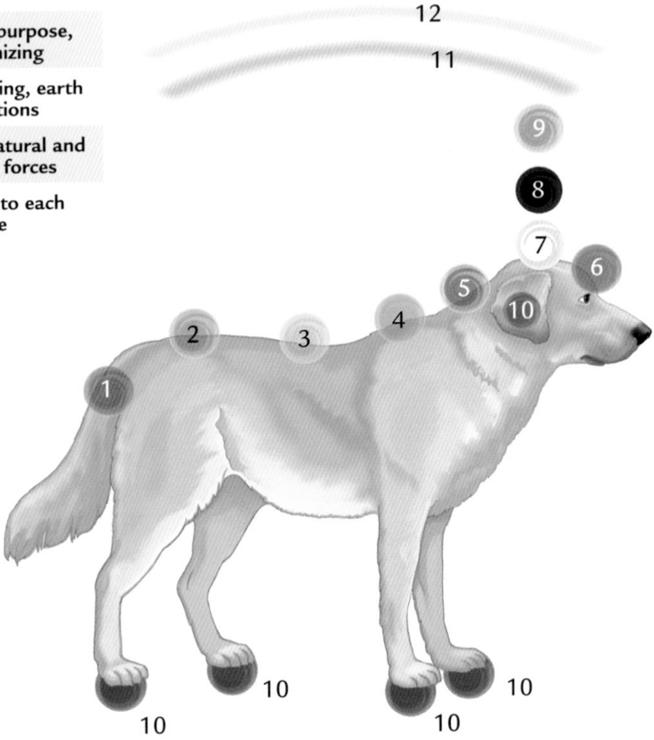

Figure 2: Mammal Chakras' Spinal and Out-of-Body Locations

The twelve chakras in all mammals, including rodents, are in the same bodily sites. This image showcases the locations of the seven in-body chakras in the spine and the five out-of-body chakras. The bud chakras are part of the tenth chakra. They are located under the ear area and under the feet. The bud chakras enable perception of environmental vibrations and noises.

Chakra	Color	Organ/Tissue
1	red	adrenals
2	orange	ovaries, testes
3	yellow	pancreas
4	green	heart
5	blue	thyroid
6	violet	pituitary
7	white	pineal
8	black or silver	thyroid (also linked to shoulder blades)
9	gold	diaphragm
10	brown	bone marrow, bud chakras
11	pink	muscles, connective tissue
12	clear	connected to 21 secondary chakras

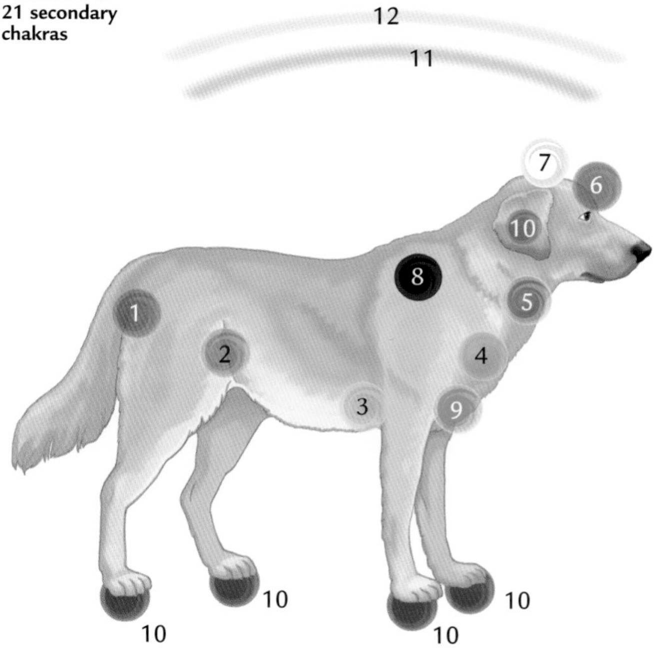

Figure 3: Mammal Chakras' In-Body Locations

This image shows the locations of the twelve chakras in relation to their major organs.

Auric Field	Color
1	red
10	brown
2	orange
3	yellow
4	green
5	blue
6	violet
7	white
8	black or silver
9	gold
11	pink
12	clear

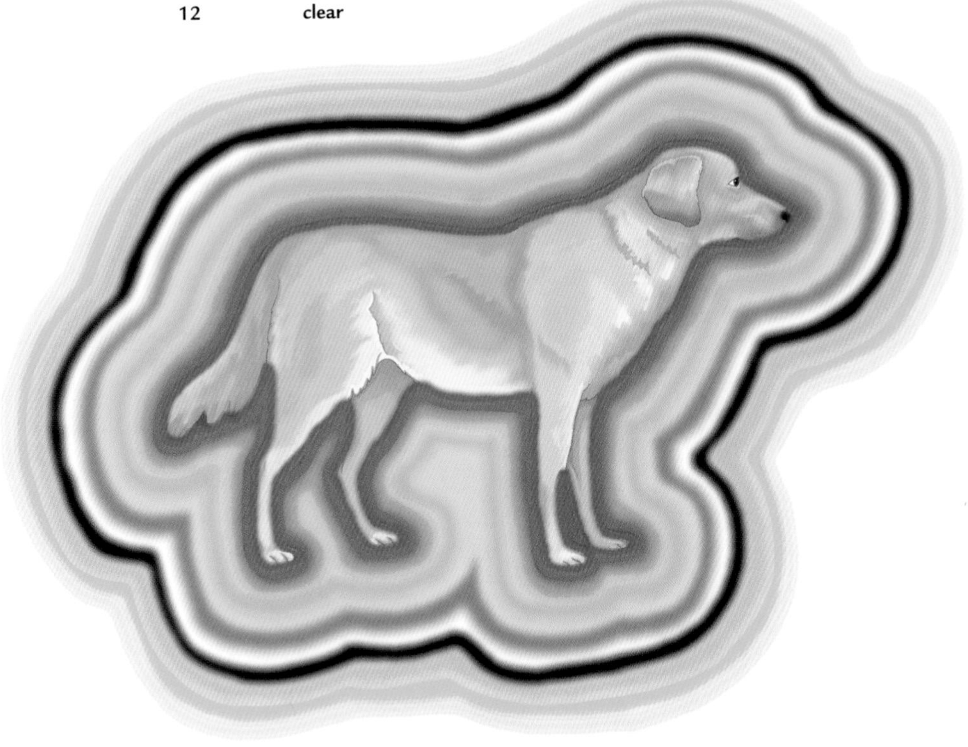

Figure 4: A Pet's Auric Field

Both humans and pets have an auric field composed of twelve individual fields. The first field begins closest to the body. The tenth field comes next and then the second; the rest proceed in numerical order.

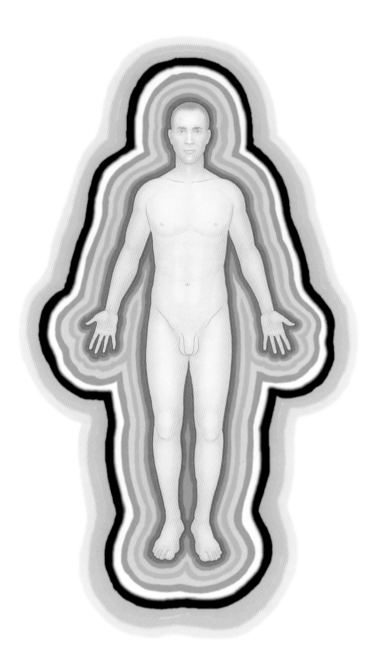

Figure 5: A Human's Auric Field

The first field is located next to the body. The tenth field comes
next and then the second; the rest proceed in numerical order
until reaching the twelfth field, which is farthest away.

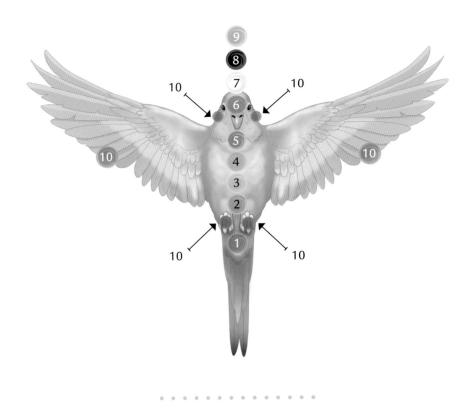

Figure 6: Bird Chakras (Front View)

This frontal view of a bird depicts the location of their twelve chakras.
A bird's tenth chakra, which includes the bud chakras, lies underneath
the claws and near the ear fissures, and includes the windtips.

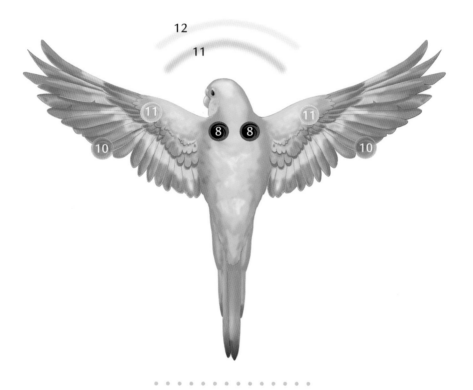

Figure 7: Bird Chakras (Back View)

This back view of a bird shows the shoulder blade region associated with the eighth chakra and the locations of the eleventh and twelfth chakras. The eleventh is outside of the body as well as linked with the bird's muscles.

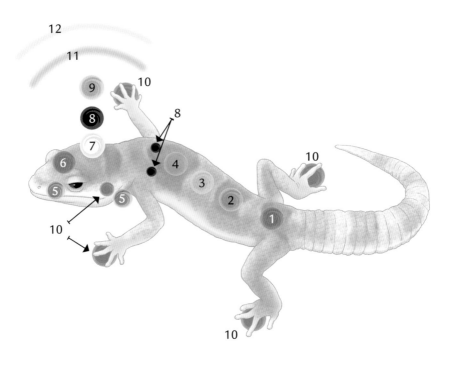

Figure 8: Lizard and Other Reptilian Chakras

This shows a lizard's twelve chakras and is representative of other reptiles and most amphibians. Because they are vertebrates, the chakras in reptiles and amphibians are similar in location to those found in mammals.

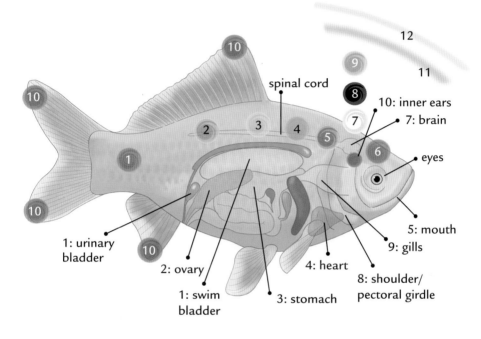

10

9

8

spinal cord

12

11

10: inner ears

7: brain

7

2

3

4

5

6

eyes

1

10

5: mouth

9: gills

10

1: urinary
bladder

10

2: ovary

4: heart

8: shoulder/
pectoral girdle

1: swim
bladder

3: stomach

Figure 9: Fish Chakras

Several organs are labeled to help you locate the chakras. Some of them are labeled with the chakra and some are independent of the chakras. In a fish, there are three parts to the tenth chakra: the fins (locomotion), the inner ears or internal bones (assess noise), and the lateral lines (these react to vibrations). The bud chakras, part of the tenth chakra, are most associated with fins.

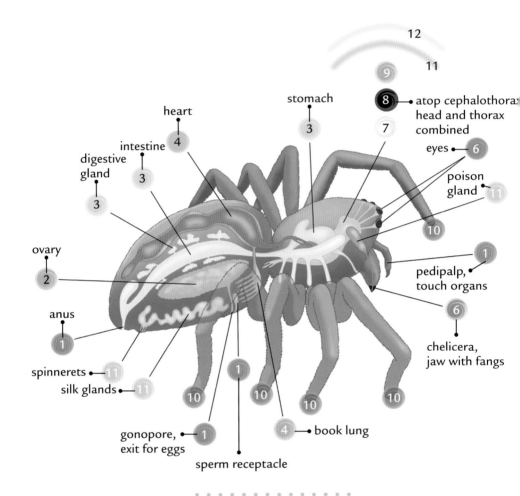

Figure 10: Chakras in Spiders and Other Invertebrates

The chakras of spiders and other invertebrates are hard to locate. Because of this, the chakras are labeled in association with their main organs. The legs are part of a spider's tenth chakra, the ends of which constitute the bud chakras. The eleventh chakra, which allows a spider to command forces through the production of venom and silk, includes bodily areas such as the spinnerets, silk glands, and poison gland.

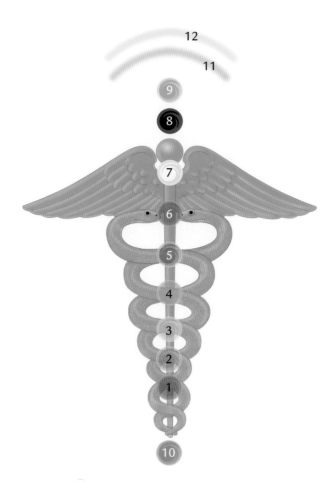

Figure 11: Chakras in a Snake

This illustration shows the location of a snake's chakras upon a caduceus, the symbol of medicine. The staff represents the sushumna nadi and the two snakes characterize the ida and pingala nadis, which are explained in this chapter. Shown are all twelve chakras. The bud chakras, part of the tenth chakra, comprise the entire underbelly.

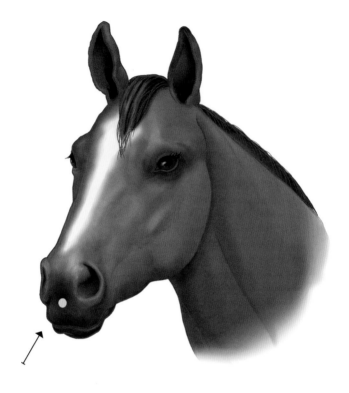

Figure 12: The Location of the Shock Acupoint

Governing Vessel 26 (GV-26), indicated by the pink dot in the illustration, can be pressed to reduce stress and release shock. It is found between the nose and the upper lip in mammals and rodents and the equivalent areas in other pets.

Chakra-by-Chakra Analysis of Challenging Issues

In order to arrive at solutions for pet problems, as well as pet/human challenges, it's easiest to link a symptom with a chakra. Eliminating issues through a chakra is an elegant and powerful process. The following chart organizes symptoms by chakras as per physical, psychological, behavioral, and spiritual signs of disharmony.

CHART: *Chakra-Based Physical, Psychological, Behavioral, and Spiritual Issues*

Chakra/ Stage	Physical Symptoms	Psychological Symptoms
First/ Survival	Overall poor health or life and death issues; skin problems; tailbone and lower hip troubles; life-threatening addictions; inflammation anywhere in body; life-threatening microbial issues; reproductive or elimination problems; adrenal and kidney disorders; some breeding issues; constant physical accidents, illnesses, or mishaps.	Issues reflecting abandonment, being unwanted, and the shame, rage, and terror that results from early rejection or abuse. Also panic attacks.
Second/ Socialization	Problems in abdominal area, such as small intestine, ovaries, testes, and sacral vertebrae. Some breeding issues, such as infertility or becoming pregnant too often.	Issues related to bonding, connection, creativity, and enjoyment of the five senses.
Third/ Learning	Poor digestion, eating disorders, and diabetes; any disorder with the gallbladder, liver, stomach, pancreas, part of esophagus, spleen, kidneys, and lumbar vertebrae. (Shares kidney disorders with first chakra.)	Issues corresponding to dysfunctional beliefs related to self-esteem and self-confidence; judgmentalism, over-opinionated; over-abundance of anxiety, fears, and worries.
Fourth/ Relating	Problems with heart, breast, ribs, pericardium, chest, upper back and blood; also cardiovascular disorders. Shoulder and arm issues can be extensions of the fourth chakra.	Issues about love, lovability, self-value, and deservedness, especially as related to healing.
Fifth/ Communicating	Reactions to noise; problems with the jaw, teeth, hearing, thyroid, throat, cervical vertebrae, neck, and parts of esophagus.	Issues related to self-expression and responsiveness to others' verbal commands and needs.
Sixth/ Self-Awareness	Issues with hormones, the pituitary, lower brain, upper spinal area, hypothalamus, eyes, and eyesight.	Issues related to self-image, self-awareness, and comparison of self with others.
Seventh/ Spiritualization	Challenges related to sleep and mood; also the pineal gland, higher thinking, top of the head, cranial bones, cerebral cavity, and cerebral plexus.	Issues about relationship with the Spirit, personal spirituality, and higher concepts such as truth, hope, and love.

Behavioral Symptoms	Spiritual Symptoms
Hyperactivity, pushiness, intense fear or rage, startle reflex, serious neediness (won't leave owner physically alone), or the opposite—lethargy, pulling away, hiding, insecurity.	Pet can absorb or express others' physical illnesses, maladies, and sensations.
Emotional eruptions, withdrawal, or obvious jealousy; intense nervousness upon not pleasing another; also lack of innovation or the opposite, trying too many new things.	Pet can absorb or reflect others' feelings, emotional problems, and second chakra physical maladies.
Acts obviously worried, edgy, nervous; displays Obsessive Compulsive Disorders (OCD) or Attention Deficit Disorder (ADD); lack of self-esteem and self-confidence or the opposite, pride and overt self-focus. Might also throw temper tantrums or refuse to represent rights.	Pet can absorb or express others' thoughts, beliefs, worries, anxieties, learning issues (a human's ADD, OCD, etc.), and third chakra physical disorders.
Attachment disorders, such as over- or under attachment and bonding; clinginess or mischievousness. Pays too much attention to ill, sick, or sad humans or other pets.	Pet can absorb or emanate higher spiritual emotions, such as appreciation, truth, and gratitude, but also beliefs of separation, lack of lovability, and more. Pet might also lose its own energy to heal others, especially assisting with others' fourth chakra maladies.
Over- or under-expressiveness; argumentativeness; inability to follow marching orders; over-eating or refusal to eat. (Too much "munching" often covers anxieties or lower chakra problems.)	Pet can absorb or reflect others' psychically verbal thoughts or desires. Can also be too open to psychic messages from others, including entities, or might completely block them out.
Behavioral excesses, self-centeredness, acts embarrassed or flaunts; also balance and coordination issues.	Pet can absorb, deflect, or mirror others' psychic impressions or self-image.
Actions related to mood disorders, such as anxiety, depression, and sleep dysfunctions; seeming inability to reason or grasp higher concepts. Pet might also show a strong sense of right and wrong, including what it or a human companion should or shouldn't do.	Pet can absorb or reflect others' sense of spiritual purpose and relationship with Spirit.

Chakra/ Stage	Physical Symptoms	Psychological Symptoms
Eighth/ Karmic Selection	Problems in shoulder blade region, with the thymus, or with chronic illness; autoimmune disorders; prevalence of entity attachments creating physical challenges. This chakra is complicit when pet displays multiple addictions, congenital disorders, and extreme problems from birth on.	All karmic issues originate in this chakra, including those that are psychological. Most prevalent psychological dysfunctions will involve at least some eighth or karmic chakra influences.
Ninth/ Dharmic Selection	Problems with breathing apparatus/ diaphragm.	Issues related to harmony and idealization. Problems will reflect deep unworthiness or superiority to others.
Tenth/ Programming	Problems with bones, stem cells, regular cells, genes, epigenetics, lower part of the ear, and the part of the pet touching the ground, such as a paw or claw; also gills in fish or wings in birds. Other signs are allergies to environmental energies and inorganic foods.	Issues reflect a pet's sense of self in the environment. Pet might shy away from the outdoors or other natural beings; hide during storms or environmental turbulence; or be aggressive with other pets or natural beings.
Eleventh/ Supernatural Powers	Problems with muscles, connective tissue, or lymph system; issues with physical movement, locomotion, and coordination.	Issues reflect comfort with using power over natural and supernatural forces. Pet can appear overly bossy, mean, punishing, or the converse, such as apologetic and meek.
Twelfth/ Transformation	Problems in any secondary chakra site, which are listed in chapter 3.	Issues reflect ability to claim the authentic and unique self and the right to activate hidden powers. Pet might appear overly meek and mild or too ambitious and scared when focused on.

Behavioral Symptoms	Spiritual Symptoms
Displays behaviors from past lives; acts opposite of how others are acting; "jumps the gun," meaning behaviors predate a future event. The pet's soul might show up in a human's visions, dreams, or intuitive faculties.	Eighth chakra gifts cross the past, present, and future. The pet can exhibit spiritual and intuitive gifts from across realms, such as bilocation or performing spirit visitations. Quite frequently, the pet will absorb nearly all of a human companion's problems to help heal them.
Over-concern with harmonizing or making everyone get along; inability to settle or be still.	Pet might take on others' ideals and desire to please them, as well as their spiritual goals. Can also lose energy to support others' spiritual goals.
Over-responsive to beings or events in environment or surroundings; actions predictive of what will occur in environment, such as becoming unsettled before an earthquake or storm.	Pets might be oversensitive to elements or love being outside. They could also exhibit a fear of the outdoors and lots of environmental sensitivities, which reveals they are taking in too many energies from the habitat.
Under- or over-performance. Pet's slight movements might result in huge disturbance of objects or the immediate environment. Sudden appearance or clearing of bad weather when the pet is around.	Pets can inadvertently attract strong natural forces or send them at others; same with supernatural forces, thus causing serious paranormal disturbances in environment.
Behaviors will reflect a pet's individual spiritual gifting.	This chakra contains a pet's individual and unique spiritual gift. Most of the time, the spiritual challenge involves a lack of gift activation or an inappropriate use of it once the pet has died, i.e., the human companion might be frightened if the pet's soul reaches out via this gift in the afterlife but has no control over it.

ed in the chakra-by-chakra analysis, by discussing the energetic conditions
involving pets in need of rescue, and by meeting Rover the rescue dog.

Understanding the Pet That Needs Rescuing

Worldwide, the plight of abandoned and unwanted animals is sadly disturbing. If an animal makes its way into a shelter, its chances of being euthanized
are high. And there are millions upon millions of needy animals requiring res-
cuing and a home. This issue is especially overwhelming if we're wondering
whether we ought to bring one of these souls into our home through fostering
or adopting, or maybe we've already experienced a rescue animal and are in full
realization of the challenges this experience promises.

Before introducing you to Rover, our case study for the energetics involved
in pet rescue, I want to lay the energetic groundwork. All new pets require
energetic support, but the rescued pet will be adversely affected by specific
energetic problems that accrue starting the very second that they are lost, given
away, turned in to a shelter, or born into homelessness. They also require special treatment if fostered, as does the human parent who will eventually give up
the fostered pet.

In all four causal situations—being lost, given up, sheltered, or born into
homelessness—the victimized pets are always affected by traumatizing forces,
many of which will be missing forces. A missing force is one of the most elusive
of traumatic injuries to assist a pet with, as it's hard to make up for what hasn't
been given: namely, safety and support. As you might expect, the pet must also
be assisted through first and fourth chakra issues, which relate to safety and
love.

Almost everyone who has rescued a pet is shocked by the multitude of emotional upheavals and behavioral disturbances. These can be off-putting but are
far easier to deal with if tracked to the related chakras and negative forces. For
instance, if a rejected animal has been kicked when on the street, it will have
a physical force impacting it and, more than likely, a resulting set of microbial
infections. If the animal has been yelled at, it will have fifth chakra difficulties.
Perhaps the pet might always whine, complain, or bare its teeth when endan-
gered. Attachments also might be involved if an original owner was kind or

loving and the abandoned animal might not want to give up that bond. As well, early childhood or past life issues might reveal some of the situations as karmic and therefore deep-seated.

To better explore this vital issue of rescue pets, which are usually cats and dogs, let's briefly look at the four situations that create the need and how they energetically impact the victimized animals.

Lost Animals

At least once a week, I spy a sign for a missing dog. By the time an advertisement is up, that pet is already stricken with missing forces as a result of feeling abandoned. It doesn't matter if the pet was the one that ran away, perhaps to chase a bunny or a whim. When an animal can't sense its human companion, the animal assumes it's been abandoned. The pet might now incur additional traumatizing forces, depending on the circumstances. Climactic hardships deliver environmental forces and injure the tenth chakra. If attacked by a coyote, a member of its own species, the missing dog might start copying the wild animal's qualities, and later, when found, lose some of its ability to show loyalty and friendliness, a dog's normal energetic signature traits. Infections can also set in, and any cords connecting the animals with its human can feel strained and stretched, leading the human to bodily and emotionally experience the conditions undergone by the lost animal.

Ironically, an attachment can actually help a pet find an owner if either are able to intuitively track it. As a human, this means that you must trust your intuition and follow it if you're searching for a lost pet.

If an accidentally lost pet finds its way home, you'll experience a few days of jittery behavior. You'll especially want to make up for the missing force by heaping a lot of love and understanding on your pet and using the other tools discussed in the remainder of this book. Some pets, however, don't vanish coincidentally.

I have a client whose father left her dog on the outskirts of town as a way to get rid of him. The father pretended that the dog had run away. Somehow, Boxer made his way home, full of cuts and burrs. Though my client, then a young girl, kept compensating for the missing force by tending to Boxer as best she could, his sense of trust was gone. He shook for months, having lost his sense of security. The techniques in this book could have instilled him with calm and eventually restored him. Unfortunately, my client was a young girl and didn't know how to care for Boxer. He became aggressive as a way of pushing off the tragedy and was put down.

Pets Given Away

Sometimes a pet doesn't work out or circumstances change and a pet is given away to a new household. A second baby, unexpected stress, a death—all kinds of situations can require the search for a new owner. Typically, this action is easier on the pet than if it's dropped off at a shelter, which we'll discuss next, but challenging energetic wounds are sustained nonetheless. Of necessity, these will include those always involved in a rescue situation, including a missing force.

In fact, the energetic damage starts as soon as the owner starts to think about giving away the pet. As already explained, pets are extremely intuitive. A pet's first chakra will immediately sense that their home life is becoming unsteady or will disappear. The missing force, even the hint of one, upsets the first chakra. This could cause the pet to get into accidents or become sick. The first chakra is primal and as the pet's primitive security is being threatened, its body will respond with physical hardships. Because of the emotional breakage, the pet might establish a cord through its fourth chakra with its current owner, which will only make the resulting change of household more disturbing when it happens. As well, the upcoming loss of structure, sensed through the pet's third chakra, will cause anxiety. Unfortunately, the resulting alteration in behavior can make it even more likely that the owner will want to get rid of the pet.

After the pet is given away, a cord can remain active. Ironically, this cord can actually cause the pet to search for its previous owner, even running away to do so. I have a great story in this regard. The first Honey the Golden Retriever, which belonged to my ex-husband when he was younger, was given to a different home once all the boys went to college. It was about twenty miles away. After one night with his new owners, Honey I escaped and ran to his previous home, arriving about mid-morning at the old homestead. He wagged his tail, ate, and was driven back, only to never leave again. I believe he'd actually erased his own cord by revisiting his previous owners. After making sure everyone was okay, he stayed away.

You'll be able to use the techniques taught in the rest of this book to support a giveaway pet, whether you're releasing it to another home or receiving it. Just remember how sensitive pets are. They'll know what's up no matter what. Because of this, common sense can be quite helpful. If possible, get the new owner together with the pet before the transfer occurs. Let everyone get to know each other and the transition will be much smoother. I was able to do this for a dog I rescued from the Humane Society. Molly had been a farm dog and never adapted to the suburbs. In fact, she could jump all the fences in the neighborhood and did so quite often. My house painter got to know her—and loved her. He would take her hunting and to his farm. It was natural for him to adopt Molly, who continued to stay with me whenever she needed babysitting.

Turned In to a Shelter

One of the most common ways that a rescued pet makes its way into a new home is through a shelter. You'll have the same energetic issues affecting this pet as in a given-away situation but additional and unique ones as well. Basically, the shelter causes its own energetic problems.

In terms of the missing forces, the effects will be aggravated. Basically, the pet was not wanted, and it might not become wanted. Consequently, the animal might try to bond with someone at the shelter, but most shelter staff members aren't available for that, leaving the pet even more emotionally wounded.

Then there is the fact that most shelters are kill shelters. This fact is terrifying to the animal on the unconscious level. At the very least, the energetics of a possible death spins the pet's seventh chakra. Any former traumas and forces will also trigger as the pet is in a life-and-death situation, although these might be repressed if the animal wants to act appropriately in order to obtain a new owner.

If you take a pet home from a shelter, know that most likely, every chakra will be stricken. Basically, any physical or emotional issues that were present or repressed when the pet was in the shelter will get triggered in your home. You'll be busy! Your new pet might also try to cord you to establish a sense of safety. Know too that in the shelter your pet might have acquired other pets' energies or a few dark forces, which you'll have to clear. You'll learn how to accomplish all these goals in this book.

A special note: If you work in a shelter, I'd suggest you learn the processes and techniques covered in chapter 8 in order to assist the souls of the euthanized pets to the other side. A single person with energetic knowledge can make a great difference for the soul of the dying animal.

Homeless Since Birth

During my many travels, often overseas, I have been struck by the plight of homeless animals. It's easy to tell that they have never had a home. The animals, which are usually cats or dogs, are skinny, unkempt, and often feral. They aren't quite wild animals, however, as the ones I've come across interact with and often depend on humans to survive.

For instance, I was recently in Marrakech and saw dozens of homeless animals, mainly cats, in the street market. Each hung out in their own area, where it seemed that they were sometimes fed by residents or stall owners. As a tourist, I found myself snagging food from the stands so I could dole out tidbits to my favorite kitties.

It is doubtful that an animal born into homelessness can become the normal "pet," a Fido the dog or Spot the cat. The missing first chakra force might be too hard to compensate for, as might the tenth chakra, which is affected by the environment. If you're tending to a homeless animal, you'll want to use the "Chakra-by-Chakra Analysis" in chapter 6 to figure out what to do. Basically, you'll stick to fixes addressing the tenth and first chakras. In fact, I have a sister who did just this with a feral cat. She knew she couldn't establish deep emotional bonds as the patterning wasn't present in the cat, which she and her girls called "Garage Kitty." The cat was never interested in coming into the house, but it would use the garage during a storm (tenth chakra) and eat the food they left out (first chakra).

If you yearn to assist the homeless-since-birth population and can't do so personally, I encourage you to volunteer for or give money to a helpful organization. Since being in Morocco, I assist Comme Chiens et Chats and follow them on Facebook. The world has become digitalized, and our ability to care for animals has as well.

When Fostering

There are special costs and gains afforded the foster parent and the pet in this temporary situation, which could at first glance be compared to a shelter. However, a foster home is anything but a shelter.

First off, the expectation is for bonding between the human and pet, which is usually a dog. In fact, one of the main tasks of the foster parent is to connect with the traumatized animal so it's ready for a deeper and more permanent bond. The other is to assist in generic training, such as to address first chakra behaviors or fifth chakra noise. These goals aren't applicable to the animal in the shelter. In becoming so personally involved with the foster pet, the human puts their heart on the line, knowing that they must eventually disconnect.

This job can be easier if the foster parent understands that they are really an energy healer. From an energetic point of view, the foster parent is actually transforming each of the animal's chakras. They might help a dog's fifth chakra by teaching them how to use their "indoor voice." They might address sixth chakra self-image problems by helping them know themselves as deserving of attention. And of course, the foster parent will be tending to first chakra physical wounds and microbial infections. The reward is an animal prepared for its forever home—like Rover, our rescue dog, who might not have been fostered but certainly needed love and care.

Rover the Rescue Dog

I met Rover's new human companion shortly after she'd obtained Rover from a shelter. Rover was a mix with so many lineages it was difficult to figure out what to call him. I'll leave you to picture a blend of Chihuahua and Chocolate Labrador.

Rover had been turned in to the same Humane Society twice, and all the records said was that he was unmanageable. When Callie, my client, adopted him, she was sure she had what it took to calm the five-year-old down.

I visited Rover at Callie's home. She looked like the mom of a not-sleeping infant. Her hair was frazzled, her clothes dirty, and she was ready to topple over. Apparently Rover never stopped moving. Ever.

As you'll learn how to do in the next chapters, I used several techniques to track Rover's various issues. I knew that his energy signature would include dog traits such as friendliness and loyalty, but also that dogs require an anchor for their fidelity. Obviously, Rover had never been bonded with; therefore, he didn't know how to accomplish this goal. My intuitive faculties showed me that he'd been rejected from conception onward, perhaps because of his mixed blood-line, and his antics suggested he had never had a first-chakra bond with a person either.

From a chakra point of view, Rover presented a couple of other interesting traits. His lack of harmony suggested a disturbed ninth chakra, which relates to soul issues. In fact, using the techniques for performing animal communication in chapter 4, I saw that he'd experienced several past lives in which he'd been rejected or unloved. These karmic undertakings also indicated a lot of eighth and tenth chakra disturbances. Rover's lack of self-knowledge also indicated a twelfth chakra issue. Plain and simple, Rover didn't know himself and wouldn't until he felt loved and wanted.

How did I help Callie? I'm going to preempt the remaining chapters and give you a hint. The missing force is always the main concern in a rescue dog. I simply worked through Rover's fourth chakra with healing streams, connecting him to Callie in a loving way. After that, she was able to meet his many physical and emotional needs because he knew he was loved.

In the end, rescue situations always start and end with love. In some ways, we could say that they are the perfect recipients of a book like this, for this is essentially a book about how to love your pet and let them love you back.

As you can see, in order to help a pet with their behavioral, psychological, physical, and spiritual challenges, it's vital to understand pet problems from an energetic point of view. This chapter laid the groundwork for following chapters. After reading a discussion about the ease with which subtle energy is transferred, you explored the nature of trauma, which is the core reason for all pet and pet/human trials. You also dug into the subtle energetics of emotions, attachments, and microbes, and you were presented with a chart listing the symptoms of pet problems chakra by chakra. And you learned about the many challenges of the rescue pet while helping out with Rover.

You are now ready to work with the data provided thus far. You'll learn about energetic solutions for your pet's various challenges.

Chapter Six
Energetic Solutions That Create More Well-Being

*No one can feel as hopeless as
the owner of a sick goldfish.*
Kin Hubbard

Our pet's troubles can leave us feeling hopeless. Of course, you'll take your pet to the vet, if applicable, and follow marching orders. The good news is that subtle energy solutions greatly expand your healing toolkit and give you reason to hope.

In a way, all previous chapters were preparatory for this one. Within this chapter you'll conjoin your knowledge of subtle energy, chakras, signatures, and pet communication to tackle your pet's behavioral, psychological, spiritual, and disease-based problems. If you're complicit in your pet's issues, the activities will also help you change and grow.

First, you'll learn how to pinpoint the origin of a pet's challenge by conducting an energetic assessment. You can reuse this assessment over and over; in fact, it's designed to be employed every time your pet exhibits an issue. After that, you'll be taught several topic-specific exercises, applying the assessment to clear karmic programs, activate dharmic energies, release cords and holds, sweep the trauma pathway, heal emotions, and transform microbes. I'll also present a section providing chakra-by-chakra tips to assist you in exploring the deeper issues embedded in each chakra. As a final bonus, I'll also suggest ways to deal with your own involvement in a pet's disorders. Overall, this chapter will bolster your capacity to assist and love your pet no matter what it's experiencing.

But before jumping in, I want to introduce you to Selma, an awesome pig that once needed subtle assistance.

The Case for a Chakra-Based Analysis

A few years ago, my client Fred introduced me to Selma, his Vietnamese pot-bellied pig. Selma had achieved the average weight of a miniature pig, about 100 pounds, and sported a little potbelly and a plump face. About a year after our first meeting, Fred called, concerned about Selma. For the past few months, she had been steadily losing weight. My assistant set up an appointment for the two of them, instructing Fred to bring laboratory reports with him.

While Selma poked around my office, I reviewed the test results, which showed that the protein levels in Selma's kidneys were slightly low. Selma was scheduled for additional tests for further exploration. In the meantime, Fred was interested in seeing what we could come up with.

Kidneys relate to the first and third chakras, as you learned in chapters 3 and 4. The first chakra, which is physical in nature and governs survival, employs the fire element. The third chakra rules mentality and willpower, displays issues related to learning, and operates through the air element. These few facts helped me create questions for delving into Selma's history, as well as Fred's life.

I started with first chakra concerns. Had Fred recently changed Selma's diet, his own, or both? Had either or both of them been physically injured or undergone a security-based loss? Yup! Right before Selma started slimming down, Fred had been demoted at work. Anything governing security issues, including a person's finances and career, relates to the first chakra. The low protein count? As you'll learn in page 162's section "Chakra-by-Chakra Practices," protein represents strength. Selma was sending first chakra power to Fred, most likely through a cord, which was depleting her own nutritional needs.

Using my intuition—and processes in this chapter—I communicated with Selma's soul and discovered that she had corded to Fred for two main reasons. First, her energetic signature, from a dharmic point of view, set her up to be caring and giving. Second, she'd experienced abandonment as a piglet. In fact, we were dealing with an empty pathway, a type of trauma induced when a pet doesn't receive what it needs during a specific stage. With this knowledge, I sent healing streams to release the cord between Fred and Selma, heal Selma's traumatized self, and activate the inner wheel of her first chakra, letting the power of that spiritual energy complete her healing. Within a month, Selma's weight and protein count normalized.

Fred also started paying more attention to Selma. He was also offered a new—and better—job in a different company. As explored in chapter 2, the energetic signature of pigs includes prosperity consciousness. *Good work, Selma!* I thought to myself. When we assist our pet, we frequently receive a personal benefit. All in all, subtle energy work served both Selma and Fred.

Before you learn how to perform the same types of maneuvers for your pet, you have to perform an energetic assessment.

Exercise
Assessing the Cause of a Pet's Problem

Solving an energetic issue starts with pinpointing the chakra or chakras that best reflect the problem's cause. This process isn't as difficult as it might seem. Chakras operate logically, as do their corollary auric fields. Since the memory of every traumatic experience is stored within the chakra that matches the related frequency, you can use the information in chapters 3 and 4—and your intuition—to identify the chakra underlying a problem.

In this two-part exercise, I'll walk you through an energetic assessment to isolate the major causal chakra. You can also focus on two chakras, but working with more than two chakras is challenging. This means you'll work with each of the two causal chakras one at a time. If there are multiple chakras involved in an issue and you can't decide which one to focus on, select either the fourth or eighth chakra. These two chakras are interactive with all the other chakras, so energies shifted through either chakra can alter all other chakras.

Specifically, the fourth chakra lies in the center of the chakra system and collects the energies from the chakras above and below it. The eighth chakra holds the intuitive knowledge of all the other chakras and can access them for psychic communication purposes. Select the fourth chakra if you believe relationship issues are involved in a challenge, and the eighth chakra if mystical or soul issues are primary.

The first of the featured stages will employ your logic, and the second will use your intuition. The third stage involves using Spirit-to-Spirit to arrive at the causal chakra/s. This assessment is key to deciding which of the many techniques featured in this chapter you'll want to apply. I encourage you to use this assessment for any and all pet concerns and before you perform any healing work.

> **1: Prepare.** To best keep track of your process, gather writing instruments. Write down your pet's presenting symptoms and your current ideas about the cause. You'll then conduct an assessment in three stages.
>
> **2: Conduct Spirit-to-Spirit.** Affirm your spirit and your pet's spirit. Also acknowledge the assistance of the invisible spirits and the Spirit.
>
> **3: Stage One, Assess Logically.** Use your mind to query about the following factors, writing down your observations.
>
> > • Assess Physical Symptoms: Is there a bodily area most affected by your pet's challenge? If so, which chakra/s serve this area? If your pet has an eye disorder, you'll select the sixth chakra. If it has digestive issues, you'll choose the third chakra.
> >
> > • Evaluate Behavioral Issues: If the pet has clear behavioral problems, pinpoint the related chakra/s. For instance, if your pet's discomfort is expressed verbally, select the fifth chakra. If the furniture magically moves when your pet is upset, isolate the eleventh chakra.
> >
> > • Analyze Psychological Challenges: If the symptoms involve feelings and beliefs, track them to the originating chakra/s. Consider the following factors.
> >
> > > *Exhibition of Obvious Psychological Issues.* For instance, if the pet is scared when you leave it alone, you're probably dealing with an abandonment issue that relates to the first chakra. If it always cowers around other pets, the issue involves personal power, which is a third chakra problem.

Issues Triggered Within You. Do you experience a specific emotional reaction when around your pet, especially in relation to its presenting issue? This could indicate the presence of an attachment or a past-life relationship between the two of you. Zoom in on which chakra/s matches your triggers. For instance, if you find yourself shouting when your pet is challenged, select the fifth chakra.

Settings That Upset the Pet. Are there particular settings or events that set off your pet? Clarify which chakra/s might relate. For instance, if your pet reacts around water, you'll focus on the second chakra, which relates to the water element.

Background Data. Consider the stories you know about your pet. Was it abused when young? Was it not fed appropriately in the last household? Was it the runt of its familial circle? Are you aware of any of the pet's past lives? All of this data can help you pinpoint a causal chakra, especially if the symptoms track with a chakra's stage of development.

- Gauge Spiritual Interactions: Are there spiritual energies or interactions that point to a specific chakra? For instance, if your pet is only in pain when you are, focus on the first chakra, the home of physical empathy. If their eyes wander under stress, look at the sixth chakra. If it seems like past-life issues are involved, select the eighth chakra.

Spend a few minutes summarizing your findings. Do all paths point to a specific chakra or a couple of chakras? You'll further hone your discoveries in the next assessment step.

4: Stage Two, Assess Intuitively. Attune your intuition with Spirit-to-Spirit and consider the following:

- Check Your Logic: Reflect on the chakra/s you found complicit in stage one. Request that the Spirit confirm your conclusions as accurate or not. You'll sense, hear, see, or feel a response. If your previous ideas weren't correct,

you'll want the Spirit to highlight the precise chakra/s
to interact with. You might psychically envision or hear,
sense, or become aware of the Spirit's answer. If there is a
difference between logic and intuition, trust your intuition.

- **Ask Your Pet:** Employ the pet communication skills you
acquired in the last chapter. Ask your pet if it believes its
challenges relate to the chakra in mind. If the pet indicates
no, ask for its opinion. Open to receiving an empathic,
visual, or verbal message, and then trust it. You can always
check with your own third chakra to get a "gut sense" and
see if you are understanding the information accurately.
If not, ask the Spirit to provide more information.

- **Reach a Conclusion:** Finally, connect with the Spirit and
finalize your decision about which chakra/s to focus on.
Write down your response. If multiple chakras are involved,
choose either the pet's fourth or eighth chakra as causal.

5: Stage Three, Define the Causal Trauma. Now focus on the causal
chakra. If you've selected two chakras, assess them one at a time. In
this stage you'll be asking questions of the Spirit, your pet's spirit,
or a spiritual guide. Typically, the information is clearest if received
from the Spirit or a spiritual guide. You can use whichever of the
follow-on questions are applicable to define the trauma:

- Is there a karmic patterning involved in this issue?

- What is the nature of the trauma that
caused the original wound?

- What type or types of forces were involved? (natural,
physical, emotional, verbal, spiritual, or empty)

- What is the pathway of the force? (entrance
site, lodged force, exit sites)

- What event or interaction caused the trauma?
When did it occur? (past life, in-between lives,
this life, developmental period in this life)

- What type of energy is still stuck or trapped—or missing from—the pet?

- What does the wounded self (stuck in the shock bubble) have to share about the causal situation or event?

- Are there attachments involved? (cords, holds) To whom or what do they connect?

- Are there any dark entities or forces? Of what sort?

- Are there introjections of others' energies? (physical, feeling-based, mental, relational, verbal, visual, environmental, forces, or others)

- Does the pet have any stuck emotions? (feelings, beliefs) What are the feelings and beliefs complicit in the problem?

- Is it important to know what's occurring in the related auric field? If so, what is happening there? Would it be helpful to work on the auric field rather than in the chakra when it's time to improve matters? (If you do need to work on the auric field, simply follow all chakra-based instructions but focus on the related field.)

- Bottom line, what is the core reason that the pet feels separate from—and therefore unworthy—in relation to the Spirit?

- What are the karmic learnings the pet's soul is seeking through this situation?

- What are the dharmic or higher results that can be achieved by facing and working through this situation?

- Is there a similar or comparable issue within me, the human companion?

6: *Summarize.* Summarize all the information obtained to select the causal chakra/s creating the problem. You'll choose ways to work on the issues as this chapter proceeds.

7: *Close.* Thank the Spirit, the guides, and your pet's spirit for all the assistance. You'll now move into the healing stage.

Healing Through the Chakras

Once you've selected one or two chakras to address, you can use the following processes to enable a shift. There are several techniques and tips to choose between. You might need to perform only one or maybe all of them, depending on the issues that arose during the assessment. Keep your assessment in mind and choose between the following activities, which perform the stated objectives.

Releasing Karmic Patterns: Clears the outside wheel of a chakra, which carries the negative programs.

Activating Dharmic Truths: Encourages the spread of the spiritual qualities from the inner wheel of a chakra.

Clearing Cords and Holds: Releases attachments from your pet and others.

Clearing the Trauma Pathway: Tracks the pathway of a trauma for cleansing and renewing purposes; also frees the pet from the shock bubble. This process might also require using the next step, which involves separating emotions.

Separating Emotions: Divorces feelings and beliefs, allowing the pet to respond to the stuck feelings and transform the primary belief from one of separation to connectivity.

Transforming Microbes: Unlocks the subtle energetics within a microbial infection.

Chakra-by-Chakra Practices: In this section, I'll review every chakra and provide a quick tip for working with each. I'll also share the energetics related to each chakra's main organs and bodily parts.

All but the last item on the list, chakra-by-chakra practices, will be taught in an exercise format.

Exercise

Releasing Karmic Patterns

The outside wheel of every chakra holds our soul's karmic patterns, as well as epigenetic issues, family-of-origin challenges, and the destructive emotions and beliefs that a pet acquires as it goes through life. This short exercise will help you better understand and also wash away the energetic problems held within the problematic chakra/s.

> *1: Prepare.* Settle into a quiet place. Your pet can be present or not.

> *2: Conduct Spirit-to-Spirit.* Affirm your spirit, your pet's spirit, and the Spirit. Now focus on the chakra that arose as causal during your assessment. If you selected two chakras, attend to one chakra now and conduct the steps in this exercise a second time for the other chakra.

> *3: Activate Your Intuition.* Ask the Spirit to activate your empathic, verbal, or visual intuition so you can receive information about your pet's issue. Then allow the Spirit to wash the outer wheel of your pet's afflicted chakra with streams of grace, thus clearing the outer wheel of energies that don't serve or belong to the pet. The streams will also sweep the most offensive karmic pattern into a bubble composed of grace.

> *4: Observe the Pattern.* This pattern, held within the bubble of grace, takes shape. The related storyline emerges so you can psychically see, sense, or hear what created the pet's karmic challenge/s. The animation reveals exactly what events or circumstances caused the pattern.

> *5: Ask for Healing.* Continue perceiving the events that caused your pet's pattern even as the Spirit sends healing streams to your pet's wounded aspect. Watch or sense your pet evolve from a troubled into a healthy state. The same streams will seep into and renew the outer wheels of the focus chakra until healing energies are shared throughout the pet's body, mind, and soul.

> *6: Close.* Thank all helpful parties and return to your everyday life when ready.

Exercise

Activating Dharmic Truths

One of the quickest ways to clear old trauma and invite healing is to activate the spiritual qualities within the inner wheel of an infected chakra. Following is an exercise that will enable this healing. Your pet can be present or not. If there is more than one causal chakras, conduct the main steps of this exercise a second time for the other chakra.

> *1: Conduct Spirit-to-Spirit.* Acknowledge your spirit, your pet's spirit, and the Spirit. You can also affirm the presence of the attending spiritual guides.
>
> *2: Focus on the Inner Wheel.* Bring your attention to the inner wheel of the causal chakra. Within lies the spiritual qualities needed to cure all ills affecting this chakra.
>
> There are many ways to stimulate the energy internal to a chakra. If your pet is present, hold your hands over the chakra's bodily location. Then ask the Spirit to spread the spiritual energy within the chakra's center throughout that chakra, the affected bodily area, and the entirety of the related auric field. You can also psychically visualize the inner wheel and ask to perceive the qualities available for healing. Watch these energies spread throughout all parts of the pet's system. You might also hear the Spirit tell you the names of the spiritual qualities dormant within the inner wheel. You might be prompted to hum, sing, speak, or otherwise verbalize these qualities so that they can extend throughout the pet; you can also perform every one of these activities. Continue this step until you sense that it is complete.
>
> *3: Close.* Thank the Spirit for the assistance and observe changes in your pet over the next few days.

Exercise
Clearing Cords and Holds

It's relatively easy to clear attachments. You simply run healing streams in and through the cords and holds. These streams lovingly heal the beings involved in the attachment, encouraging all parties to address their unconscious concerns in the way healthiest to them.

However, there are two caveats involved in releasing attachments. It might be necessary to understand the reason that an attachment initially developed. If so, it's because there is a dharmic teaching that will keep your pet forever free from the attachment. The second caveat exists if the attachment links you and your pet. There might be a higher lesson for you that becomes apparent through this healing.

The following steps will assist you in releasing an attachment and also dealing with the two stipulations just mentioned, if applicable.

> *1: Prepare.* Decide if you want your pet present or not. Breathe deeply.
> Based on the assessment conducted earlier in this chapter, survey
> your thoughts. Do you think you are dealing with a cord, a hold, or
> both? What type? I'll summarize the various cords and holds in this
> exercise; for now, take a first swipe at a diagnosis.
>
> *2: Conduct Spirit-to-Spirit.* Affirm your spirit, the pet's spirit, and all
> helping spirits. Then affirm the Spirit.
>
> *3: Analyze the Attachment.* Ask the Spirit to help you further analyze
> the pet's attachment. In this step you'll be reviewing the types of
> attachments and requesting that the Spirit provide you a sensation,
> emotional reaction, thought, awareness, vision, or verbal insight
> depicting what you're dealing with. The pet might be afflicted with
> more than one attachment; ask to know about each one.
>
> • Which of the following is occurring in my pet?
>
> Cord. Causes an unhealthy flow of energy
> between one or more parties.
>
> Life Energy Cord. Forces loss of life energy in pet; this
> energy is taken by one or more external parties.

Curse. Collection of tangled energies that create negative reactions or an inability to attract positive situations.

Marker. An X that instructs the external world how to mistreat the pet.

Possession. An energetic vulnerability that allows a possessive entity to take over.

Deflection. A thin film that rejects positive energies.

- What are the nuances of the attachment?

  Where does the attachment lock into or affect my pet? (bodily area, mind, soul, chakra/s, auric field/s)

  To what or whom is the pet attached?

  In what time period was the attachment established?

  What circumstances created this attachment?

  How is this attachment negatively affecting my pet?

  What does my pet need to learn to be released from this interchange?

  If I'm personally involved, I will answer these questions:

  What part did I play in the creation of the attachment?

  What part do I play in the upkeep of it?

  How am I harming or seeking to help my pet through the attachment?

  How is the attachment seemingly benefiting or harming me?

  What do I need to understand about love to free myself and my pet?

4: Further Analyze for Entities. Ask the Spirit to reveal the presence of any dark force, entity, or interference, if any exist. If there are none present, skip this step. Then request that the Spirit reveal whether or not you should communicate with the entity (or entities) on behalf of your pet. If the Spirit shows that you should, it will surround the entity in healing streams, which form a bubble of grace. Caught in this bubble, the entity won't be able to further influence or harm the pet or you. It must, however, respond to questions. These questions, directed at the interference, can include the following:

- For what reason did you connect to the pet?
- What are you seeking to take or give the pet?
- How are you taking advantage of the pet?
- What is the storyline that created the connection?
- Are you willing to be released from the pet? What do you require to do so?

5: Apply Healing Streams of Grace. It's now time to request the healing streams. Ask the Spirit to send these to dissolve, fill in, and release all cords or holds. These streams will provide deep healing for any and all contract holders, including any entities. If a contract holder, even if it's an entity, refuses to let go, it will be lovingly taken away by the Spirit. Observe, feel, or hear these streams do their work until it's done.

6: Close. Thank all the powers that provided insight and healing and return to your everyday life when ready. Watch for the responses exhibited by your pet.

Exercise
Clearing the Trauma Pathway

There are many steps involved in energetic trauma recovery, no matter the type of force that carried in the destructive energies. Simplistically, these steps are as follows:

- find and repair entry and exit sites and unstick lodged forces
- clear out and fill in pathways
- soothe the thalamus
- liberate and reintegrate the shocked self

You'll use healing streams to achieve these goals. In the next chapter you'll be provided vibrational supports to enable a more thorough recovery. You might also need to provide further healing to the traumatized self. To do that, I indicate where to use page 158's exercise "Separating Emotions."

While this exercise aims at healing old trauma, you can also clear trauma just before, during, or after its occurrence. The tip provided right after this exercise can be used for on-the-spot trauma clearing.

1: Prepare. Your pet can be present or not. If it is, select an environment that is comfortable for both of you. If alone, select a quiet space in which to conduct this exercise.

2: Conduct Spirit-to-Spirit. Affirm your spirit, the pet's spirit, the guiding spirits, and all spirits that were involved in your pet's original trauma. Then affirm the Spirit.

3: Clarify the Trauma. Based on the assessment you conducted in this chapter, focus on the chakra that matches the trauma. If you selected two chakras, conduct this exercise twice. Now ask the Spirit to help you better understand the actual trauma. If suitable, simultaneously perform pet communication and allow yourself to receive information directly from the pet. What event wounded your pet? What type of force/s carried in the damage—natural, physical, emotional, verbal, spiritual, or empty? What kind of subtle energies were loaded into the pet's body, mind, or soul, such as physical, psychological, or spiritual?

You might actually perceive the shock bubble in which the pet's struggling self is stuck. Psychically peer through this bubble and allow yourself to directly communicate with the injured pet, collecting information even while sending love to this scared self.

4: Find the Entry Point. Still in a meditative state, ask the Spirit to reveal the trauma's entry site. You might psychically visualize it, hear a message, or feel a physical sensation, emotion, awareness, or know about the correct part of the pet's body, chakra, or auric field. Ask the Spirit to reveal how this entry point has been impacting your pet.

5: Follow the Pathway. Energetically follow the pathway caused by the invading force, becoming aware of the pathway. Is it clear, clogged, or littered with subtle energies? Might it be an empty pathway, indicative of a trauma caused by missing but needed energy? Also ask that the Spirit reveal an exit point, if there is one. Then request an understanding of how the pathway and exit point, if the latter exists, has been affecting the pet.

6: Request Healing Streams. It's now time for the Spirit to send healing streams through the entrance point, pathway, and any exit point. These streams will clear and fill the pathway.

7: Heal the Wounded Self. If you previously identified the wounded aspect of your pet, ask the Spirit to send healing streams through the shock bubble to heal the pet. The Spirit will attend to all your pet's needs.

8: Clear the Thalamus. Ask the Spirit to replace the shock bubble with healing streams and clear the thalamus, releasing the traumatized self from the bubble. This newly created enclosure of grace will assure that the wounded self grieves in a healthy way and also provides protection. It is here that you would use the exercise "Separating Emotions" on page 158 to provide further emotional assistance.

9: Close. Ask the Spirit if there are any additional tasks to perform for your pet. Return to your everyday life when ready.

Additional Tip

Clearing a Trauma Just Before, Immediately After, and While It's Occurring

What can you do if you're present during a pet's traumatic experience or even just before or after the event? The answer is to quickly conduct Spirit-to-Spirit and ask the Spirit to immediately deliver healing streams. I'm always surprised at how effective this action is.

For instance, I once watched a large bird scoop up my pet bunny when we were outside. While scaring off the bird, I also sent healing streams, from a distance, to my shaking bunny. Within a few moments he started breathing regularly, but there were puncture marks on the poor thing. I then stroked the area around the wound marks. Still requesting the Spirit's help, I simultaneously asked that healing streams be sent into the entrance wound. I could actually sense the streams moving into the entrance wound and through the pathway, then all the way beyond the energetic exit site. The wound healed within a day, although there was a tiny bump at the exit wound site that had not been there previously.

You can also use streams of grace to prepare a pet for an upcoming trauma. After all, what pet likes visiting the veterinarian, getting shots, taking medicine, undergoing surgery, traveling, or being forced to participate in some other dislikable task? For example, before I take my dogs in for their teeth cleaning, which is performed under anesthesia, I send healing streams through the entirety of my dogs' systems and also to the surgical staff. The healing streams enable a safe reaction to the anesthesia and detoxify the dogs after the event. They also keep the medical staff on-point. The only time I forgot to send the healing streams, the dogs took three days instead of a single day to get their act together post–teeth cleaning.

Exercise
Separating Emotions

As we discussed in chapter 4, emotions are composed of one or more feelings and beliefs that are stuck together. In this exercise you'll be shown how to use your pet communication skills to help your pet release intertwined feelings and beliefs, heed the messages within the feelings, and convert a negative belief into a connecting one. You'll interact with the pet's spirit as well as the Spirit.

> **1: Prepare.** Grab a paper and pen so you can keep track of the insights gained. Your pet can be present or not. Review or run through the assessment in this chapter and focus on the selected chakra. You can repeat this exercise's steps if there are multiple chakras, as different emotions can be housed in different chakras.

> **2: Conduct Spirit-to-Spirit.** Acknowledge your own spirit and that of your pet's. Then affirm the helping spirits and the spirits of any being involved in the emotional disarray. Lastly, turn the process over to the Spirit.

3: Connect with Your Pet. You will simultaneously communicate with the Spirit and with your pet's spirit. Make contact and focus on the chakra that holds the emotional issue.

4: Communicate with Your Pet. Ask your pet to help you better sense, feel, or hear about the stuck emotion that's causing problems. It is most likely that the aspect of the pet most affected by this emotion is stuck in a shock bubble. Ask to perceive that bubble, knowing that the Spirit will make it translucent so you can interact with the traumatized aspect of the pet. Let the pet share whatever it needs to about the causal event—the situation, circumstances, parties involved, and the like. Make sure your pet feels understood on all levels.

5: Subdivide the Emotion. Request that the Spirit divide the emotion into three parts, using images, senses, or sounds to reveal the percentages of energy in these categories:

- feelings
- beliefs
- others' energies

Then ask the Spirit to release the pet from the energies that don't belong to them. The resulting vacuum will be replaced with healing streams.

6: Analyze the Feelings. Ask the pet and the Spirit to relay all the pet's feelings that are causing problems. Then write down how the pet needs to honor the related feeling. For clues, refer to the data in the section "Emotions: Of Havoc and Healing" in chapter 4, and also the following list, which provides prompting questions.

- **Fear:** What needs to be done to move to safety?
- **Anger:** What boundaries need to be established and how?
- **Sadness:** What needs to be known to reclaim the truth of love?
- **Disgust:** What toxic energy must be taken away or avoided?
- **Happiness:** How does the pet get more happiness and joy?

Focus on each applicable feeling until you sense that your pet, especially its wounded self, is feeling empowered.

7: *Transform the Beliefs.* No matter the beliefs affecting the pet, if a negative belief has been chained to a feeling, it is focused on separation rather than connection. Simply ask the Spirit to present the pet with a love-based belief, which will replace any and all separating beliefs. You'll sense, hear, feel, or perceive this new and correct belief within yourself as well. Sense the transformation of your pet as well as yourself.

8: *Move to Completion.* It's time for the Spirit to flow streams of grace through the pet's affected chakra and beyond, completing the healing. These streams will help the pet respect its feelings, trust love, and release any remaining trauma. Ask that any corollary emotions within you be assisted as well, especially if any were returned to you by your pet.

9: *Close.* Thank the Spirit for the help and return to your everyday life when ready.

Exercise
Transforming Microbes

Those pesky microbes—they cause everything from annoying coughs to life-threatening illnesses. Bolster your pet's immune system, as well as any medicine prescribed by a veterinarian, by cleansing and transforming the subtle energetics involved in microbial infections. For more information about microbes, refer back to page 128's section "The Subtle Energies in Microbes."

1: *Prepare.* Review the assessment from the earlier part of this chapter and focus on the microbe causing your pet's problems. You can also employ knowledge obtained from the medical community, such as via test results. Your pet can be present or not during this process.

2: *Conduct Spirit-to-Spirit.* Acknowledge your own spirit, your pet's spirit, and the Spirit.

3: *Analyze for Cause and Situation.* Focus on the chakra related to the microbe. If there are additional microbial infections, you can conduct this exercise again with a different microbe in mind. Now review the issues laden in the afflicting microbe. As a reminder, here are hints:

- **Bacteria:** Holds pet's repressed feelings.
- **Parasites:** Mirrors forces or beings stealing energy from the pet.
- **Yeasts, Fungus, and Molds:** Same as parasites; also store others' feelings.
- **Viruses:** Parasitic but also corded to an external source, such as an entity, family system, or another living being.

Ask the Spirit to provide you additional insights about the situation linking your pet to the problematic microbe. You might psychically see, sense, feel, hear about, or perceive a response. What circumstances caused the pet to bond with the microbe? What hidden belief or emotion is making the pet unconsciously hold onto the microbe? Is there a trauma involved? If so, what needs to be known to release it? Continue to ask questions of the Spirit that flesh out the connection between the microbe and the pet. Hone your questions based on the chakra the microbe is most affiliated with, reviewing the chakra descriptions in chapters 3 and 4. For instance, if the microbe infects a bird's claws, you'll focus on the tenth chakra. If there are fleas on a dog's shoulder blades, you'll examine the eighth chakra. If a breathing issue has resulted from the microbe, choose the ninth chakra.

4: Request Healing Streams. The Spirit will now send healing streams through the chakra and bodily parts infected by the microbe. If others' feelings have been absorbed, they are now lovingly returned to the spirit they belong to. If the pet is storing its own repressed feelings, these will be stimulated in a gentle manner. If external beings or forces have been taking advantage of your pet, this situation will be alleviated and all cords and holds dissolved.

5: Close. Thank the Spirit and all the helpers for this assistance and return to your life when ready.

Chakra-by-Chakra Practices

To quickly hone in on a chakric concern, here I provide a brief summary of each chakra. Also described are the subtle energy meanings of the main organs and bodily parts associated with each chakra. Simply convert the listed body part into the closest one that pertains to your type of pet.

First Chakra

Physical movement and exercise—or, conversely, rest—will alleviate a first chakra issue. Also support the pet with healthy food. In general, there are only three basic types of nutrients, which represent the following energies:

- Proteins lend strength, fortitude, and power.
- Carbohydrates provide instant energy, brain power, comfort, and joy.
- Fats deliver enrichment and stability, and also serve as a foundational bonding material.

How might you apply the above information? Remember Selma the pig from the beginning of the chapter? She was lending her protein, or strength, to her human companion. That clue helped us pinpoint her causal issues.

In relating organs to issues, consider what first chakra organs and body parts represent.

- **Large Intestine:** Waste management and timeliness of releasing toxins.
- **Anus and Rectum:** Discharge of physical and subtle toxins.
- **Vagina:** Procreation desires and feminine sexuality.
- **Adrenals:** Fight, flight, and freeze capabilities and all stress-based reactions.
- **Kidneys:** See third chakra.
- **Bladder:** Storage of extra energy.
- **Skin:** Protection and reaction to external world.
- **Pelvis:** Decisions about moving forward.

Second Chakra

Analyze the pet for emotional health and expression. Also search your own feelings to make sure your pet isn't mirroring your emotional issues. Second chakra organs and body parts represent the following issues:

- **Small Intestine:** Separates helpful and unhelpful ideas and nutrients.

- **Ovaries and Testes:** Partnering ability; passing down of legacy.

- **Womb:** Serves as an internal universe representing the divine feminine.

- **Prostate:** Sense of adequacy.

Third Chakra

Use logic to assess third chakra concerns. Also address dysfunctional beliefs, stuck emotions, and dietary needs. The related organ and body parts are represented in the following ways.

- **Pancreas:** "Sugars" or sweetness and joys of life.

- **Liver:** Reactions to male energies and power.

- **Gallbladder:** Holds visions of the future and raging (angry and hurt) emotions.

- **Stomach:** Breaks down ideas and nutrients for assimilation.

- **Spleen:** Reactions to female energies and power.

- **Kidneys:** Also a first chakra organ, represent childhood fears and the relationship with ancestral programming.

- **Esophagus:** Also serving the fourth and fifth chakras, represents what the pet is "swallowing" that is healthy or unhealthy.

Fourth Chakra

Always examine the needs for and reactions to love. Specific body parts can represent the following ideas:

- **Heart:** Giving and receiving of love.

- **Breasts:** Relationship to maternal love.

- **Ribs:** Perceptions about the safety of love.

- **Lungs:** Ability to receive from the Spirit.

- **Cardiovascular System:** The pet's ability to share and distribute love.
- **Arms:** Extensions of the heart; grasping and releasing of desires.

For specific cardiovascular concerns, consider the symptoms. For instance, high blood pressure represents performance pressure. Low blood pressure indicates that the pet doesn't feel believed in. Vein or artery issues relate to the pet's ability to self-love.

Fifth Chakra

Assess communication issues, entity interference, and verbal treatment of the pet. Organs and their meanings include the following:

- **Thyroid:** Ability to express desires.
- **Ears:** Receiving messages.
- **Nostrils:** Management of vitality.
- **Neck:** Honoring of personal views.
- **Teeth:** Ability to express specific truths.
- **Shoulders:** Burdens being carried.
- **Sinuses:** Responses to others' psychic messages.
- **Nose:** Spiritual direction.

Sixth Chakra

Overall, assess self-image and planning abilities. Specific organs and body parts and their associations are described next.

- **Pituitary:** Vision for manifesting.
- **Thalamus:** Management of shock and obsessiveness.
- **Eyes:** Perceptions of self and others.
- **Forehead:** How the pet is facing the world.

Seventh Chakra

Attune to consciousness and spirituality, with specific organ and bodily parts representing the following:

- **Pineal Gland:** Expression of life purpose.
- **Cranium Bones:** Ability to set flexible but ethical standards.

- **Upper Brain:** Access to higher knowledge.
- **Crystals in the Brain:** Attunement to nature's cycles.

Eighth Chakra

Search the mystical planes for causes and solutions to issues and examine the following organ and body parts:

- **Thymus:** Immune function; the ability to make peace with internal and external factors and beings.
- **Shoulder Blades:** Reactions to unseen beings and forces.

Ninth Chakra

Review the soul's sense of worthiness in relation to the Spirit. The ninth chakra is represented by the diaphragm, which relates to the pet's ability to take in the Spirit's insight and support.

Tenth Chakra

Assess genetic and epigenetic matters and the pet's relationship with the natural world. Also focus on the following organs and body parts and what they mean:

- **Bones and Structural System:** Foundation of pet's beliefs and interactions with the world.
- **Ankles:** Flexibility of action.
- **Feet/Hands:** Advancement of personal self.

Eleventh Chakra

Evaluate the presence and effects of natural and supernatural forces on the muscular system. Ask if the pet is over- or under-utilizing its willpower and supernatural capabilities. In particular, the connective tissues represent connection.

Twelfth Chakra

This chakra is unique to the pet. You can examine the meaning of the secondary chakra sites, which are served by the twelfth chakra, in page 89's chart "A Pet's Twenty-One Secondary Chakras."

A few additional pointers will assist you in helping your pet.

> ***Nervous System Concerns.*** The nervous system represents communication and the flow of vital energy. Address neurological concerns by examining the pet's fundamental desire to be alive.

> ***Sides of the Body.*** In general, the left side of the body represents issues with feminine traits or females and the right side of the body relates to issues with masculine traits or males.

> ***Front and Back Sides of the Body.*** Overall, the front side of the body showcases a pet's interactions with the everyday world and their use of conscious knowledge. The back side of the body takes in unseen energies and reflects a pet's unconscious issues.

Having examined the foundational energetics of a pet's issues and the techniques needed to address them, you're now ready to explore the vibrational medicines that can make a huge difference in your pet's life.

Chapter Seven
Vibrational Medicines and Tools for Health and Well-Being

If we are beings of energy,
then it follows that we can
be affected by energy.

Richard Gerber

Vibrational medicine is an analytical and healing approach to creating balance using energetic frequencies. When balance is brought to behavioral, psychological, disease, and spiritual processes, the pet's body, mind, and soul can right itself. Because you are so interconnected to the pet, your own life will improve as well.

As we've established, the basis of all energetics—as well as everything in life—is light and sound. Light is the basis of an X-ray machine and laser technology. Ultrasound therapy utilizes sound waves to relax tissues, increase blood flow, and break down scar tissue. While measurable therapies are certainly potent, subtle therapies can be equally powerful, whether they are the "main course" or supplemental. When you alter the subtle energies underlying a physical disorder, you shift the framework causing the malady. By adding the right subtle frequencies, you bring about a healthier state.

This chapter offers a sampling of my favorite vibrational tools and practices. You can also find additional information about each concept and technique on the internet and through professional services. In fact, if you have any questions about a medicine or its application, I encourage you to engage an expert. Vibrational medicines are just that. They are medicines. Because of this, if improperly selected or delivered, they can make matters worse, not better.

Before filling your subtle energy toolkit, I want to more thoroughly explain vibrational medicines. I'll accomplish this goal by first exploring stone therapy, one of the many types of vibrational medicines covered in this chapter. I'll then introduce you to three amazing subtle experts: Royal Rife, Hans Jenny, and Björn Nordenström. Their near-miraculous research and work will prove the point that subtle energetic medicines can make a huge difference in a pet's life.

I'll then outline several processes you can employ to support your pet's well-being. These include the combined use of hands-on healing and light, an introduction to a vital acupoint, and the use of toning and music, essential oils, flower essences, homeopathy, and stone therapy.

And now, buckle up. Next stop: the vibrational frontier.

The Former and Future Frontier

Frequency-Based Healing

Since time began, healers, shamans, medics, doctors, and the like have used frequency-based tools and medicines to support living beings. The fundamental understanding is that one form of energy can alter the vibrational resonance of other forms of energy.

After giving you an example of a specific type of vibrational medicine, stone therapy, I'm going to introduce you to three of the "famous greats" in the energetic field. The purpose is to show you exactly how vibrational medicines work so that you can feel confident in your use of them.

One of the most widely accepted vibrational modalities is, and has always been, the use of crystals and other types of stones. In ancient Egypt the dead were buried with quartz on their forehead; the stone's energy guided the soul into the afterlife. Living Egyptians wore crystals over their hearts to attract love and crystal crowns upon their heads to awaken their clairvoyance.

Chinese medical practitioners used crystal-tipped needles to perform acupuncture, even while Greek soldiers were rubbing crushed hematite on their bodies to make them invincible. And named in the Christian Old Testament and the Hindu Vedic Scriptures are stones representing various sacred and healing powers. Personally, almost every culture I've visited around the world, many of them indigenous, employs some sort of stone therapy, whether the stones are laid directly on a body, sung or chanted into, consulted for information, crushed and flung into an environment, or formulated into a tincture. And these stones are used for everything from healing physical and psychological concerns to relating to spiritual guides. You'll learn more about stone therapy at the end of this chapter.

More recently, science is starting to explain how interactions with stones enable transformation. Basically, a crystal, which vibrates at its own frequency, impacts a natural being's energy field through resonance. The incoming frequencies influence the being's field but also its chakras, introducing new information into the nervous system and physical body, thus stimulating biochemical shifts. In quantum physical language, when two objects vibrate in the same space at the same time, like a stone and a dog, they affect each other. In other words, the energetic structure, light, and sound of a stone reprograms the resonant, or matching, energies of the pet (Lucas 2014).

All other vibrational medicines work in basically the same way—through resonance. But how exactly does resonance work? Take a bow, Royal Raymond Rife, our next "speaker."

Royal Rife was an American inventor who died in 1971. In the 1930s he developed a special optical microscope that could reveal microbes too small to perceive with previous technology. His hundreds of experiments showed that refracted light of various frequencies could weaken or destroy pathogens and even change a lethal microbe into a non-lethal one. The process also transformed the microbes causing cancer. His basic theory was that every disease or condition has its own electromagnetic signature. By disturbing that signature, either through delivering a frequency that has a "mortal oscillation" or altering the medium in which the microbe exists, the pathogen was eliminated.

How could this happen?

One of the theorists whose ideas explain how Rife's treatments cured disease was Mayo Clinic physician Edward Rosenow. Rosenow asserted that microbes including bacteria aren't actually lethal; rather, they are primitive forms of life that modify in response to the environment. They are therefore beneficial or malevolent depending on the conditions in the host. The conditions that invite a disease state include injury, stress, or a weakening of protection (Lee Foundation, n.d.). In other words—and here is one of our main themes—trauma alters an environment in such a way that microbes become destructive.

Rife's microscope was actually able to direct light, or bend it, in ways that proved Rosenow's views were correct. Succinctly, Rife's experiments showed that every microbe gives off a wave of ultraviolet light. To alter a microbe, he first applied another ultra-violet frequency to convert the microbe's currency into regular light. He then subjected the microbe to a specific short wave frequency that would cause the microbe to disintegrate. Furthermore, by altering the environment, including the food supply, he could shift a friendly germ into a lethal germ and vice versa. Moreover, Rife proposed ten different categories of microbes, showing how the correct frequencies of light could convert one into another (Lee Foundation, n.d.).

Energetically, I've employed these concepts to send the correct coloration and refraction of light to help heal microbial infections but also trauma in people and pets. Because I ask the Spirit to select and direct the light, I know that the frequencies are always correct. Using this technique, a human client's long-term staph infection nearly disappeared in a day, another human's neck—injured in an accident—straightened out, and a pet's parasitic condition was eliminated within a week. You'll practice this concept in the "Hands-Based Healing with Color and Intention" exercise on page 173.

So far, I've been exploring the power of light to effect change. Sound is an equally impressive force, with the potency of sound healing revealed through a discipline called cymatics, the study of visible sound, or wave vibrations. One of the first modern Western pioneers in this field was Dr. Hans Jenny, who based his work on early theories by Ernst Chladni, a German physicist and musician who lived in the mid 1750s. Jenny's experiments involved sending sound over materials such as sand, water, paste, and the like. Different sounds formed different patterns on the materials, showing that sound creates shapes that mirror but also affect the natural world (Volk, n.d.).

More recently, sounding has been scientifically proven to help people recover from stroke, surgery, chronic pain, cognitive deficits, stress, pain, headaches, and premenstrual syndrome (Wagner 2013). In this book we'll employ the sounds related to the Hindu chakra system to encourage healing in your pet.

Vibrational medicines, all of which invite a shift in light, sound, or both, can most easily be directed toward a chakra or related field. In chapter 2 we also discussed the existence of a third set of subtle structures, the energy channels. Of the nadis and the meridians, the meridians are the most easily accessible subtle channels, with meridian-based therapies in use for over 5,000 years. I believe the most grounded physical explanation of meridians was offered by Dr. Björn E. W. Nordenström, a former president of the Nobel Prize Assembly and Swedish radiologist and surgeon. Nordenström began researching the bio-electrical nature of bodily injury starting around the 1960s. Amazingly, he cured dozens of people with cancer using the same ideas we've explored in this book, also effecting change in conditions including macular degeneration, wound healing, neuropathy, retinopathy, and more (IABC, n.d.).

My personal explanation of Nordenström's theory is that the body is a closed electrical circuit composed of microcurrents. Measurable and subtle energies flow along the lines known as acupuncture meridians. In turn, these ionized energies, encapsulated in a watery tube of hyaluronic acid, send ionized charges into the cardiovascular system and then into the central nervous system. Problems set in because there is too much electricity or magnetism at the sites of an injured area. Eventually, that area begins producing its own charges, causing further disruption. In the case of cancer, a tumor is formed. Mental processes and force fields, such as healing delivered through healing hands, can alter the imbalanced energies and enable the body to heal (Natural Connections Healthcare, n.d.; Rexresearch.com, n.d.).

My summation of Nordenström's work reveals why meridian-based therapies can help release traumatic forces and subtle and physical challenges. Essentially, interacting with the meridians, usually through the acupoints, shifts the electrical and magnetic balance of an injury site. I'll show you a one-step method for releasing a pet from shock in the tip provided after the next section.

Ready to roll up your sleeves and get to work? Let's bend light with our hands—and mind—and alter a pet's well-being.

Hands-On Healing with Light

Light is a healing property. Study after study shows that specific frequencies and vectors of light affect physical reality in distinct ways. In conventional modalities, specific colors/frequencies have treated psoriasis and microbial infections, increased activity in chickens, obtained higher yields of plants, killed pesky insects, altered the mood in an environment, and more. The allopathic world is only now starting to explore the benefits of color healing, which has been used since at least the sixth century BCE. Basically, light influences every aspect of a biological system and can even be considered a form of nutrition (Altered State, n.d.).

One of the easiest ways to deliver light to a pet is through the hands, which I'll show you how to do. First, a few words on why the hands are so important.

Basically, hands are an extension of the heart chakra; specifically, the heart organ. To gain the most advantage in healing, we want to employ the natural physical and subtle energies of the heart, which is the most powerful electromagnetic organ in the body.

Compared to the brain, the heart's electrical field is 60 times greater in amplitude, and its magnetic field is 5,000 times more potent. Not only does its field permeate and affect every cell in the body, but it extends far beyond the body, interconnecting one being with another. Within and beyond the bounds of the heart's measurable field, subtle energetic exchanges affect everything from physiology to social behaviors. This psychic communication allows the heart and the brain to receive intuitive information, even from the future, and process subtle data. In fact, about 65 percent of the heart's cells are neurological, not muscular, meaning it can "think" and enable important decision making.

The interactivity of heart-based fields also means that energetic exchanges between beings are contagious. This is true of human-to-human connections but also human-animal. Moreover, the science shows that when we focus our heart on positive emotions and spiritual qualities, such as love and appreciation, rather than negative emotions and qualities, all levels of health improve. In contrast, negative energies cause illness (McCraty 2015). What this means is that holding positivity in your heart (and hands) can greatly improve your pet's well-being.

How powerful to blend the correct frequencies and vectors of light with emanations from your heart and hands! You'll be doing that in the following exercise. You can decide to touch your pet, hold your hands away from them, or simply direct a mental stream of energy at your pet. It doesn't matter; healing streams do the work.

Exercise
Hands-Based Healing with Color and Intention

This exercise will help you accomplish three goals. After selecting a pet concern, you'll compose a statement for a desirable healing, select a color related to the healing goal, and use your hands to direct healing streams of grace. It's preferable to be near your pet, but it's not necessary. All practices can be conducted within your mind's eye, as subtle energy can be sent and received at a distance.

> **1: Prepare.** Focus on the issue you'd like to help your pet with. You can use a subject that came up during the assessment in the last chapter or create a different one. Select the correlated chakra/s, auric field/s, bodily area, trauma pathway, or traumatized self. You can also direct healing energy to the entirety of a pet, an aspect of its soul, or even straight into the internal wheels of all chakras for a full activation of dharmic qualities. Now settle into a relaxed state.

> **2: Conduct Spirit-to-Spirit.** Affirm your spirit, your pet's spirit, and all helping spirits. Also acknowledge the Spirit, which will manage this healing process.

> **3: Create a Healing Statement.** Formulate a positive statement that encapsulates the desired healing. Make the phrase uplifting so it reflects positive emotions and qualities and stimulates heart-based healing. For instance, you might state, "I request that the Spirit clear the electromagnetic energies causing my pet's tumor and rebalance that bodily area." You can also formulate a generic request, such as, "I desire that the Spirit bring my pet's system into perfect harmony."

> **4: Select a Color.** Read through the following synopsis and select one or two colors to focus on. The healing energies encompassed

in each color are described. The chosen color/s will be added to healing streams in the next step and shaped into the refraction needed to achieve the healing statement.

CHART: *The Healing Energies of Colors*

Color	Healing Energies
Red	Heats, warms, purges; adds physical vitality, courage, and life energy. Addresses life-threatening issues.
Orange	Cheers, frees; separates emotions and induces positivity; enables a new response to a stuck pattern.
Yellow	Awakens, stimulates; eases the nerves and strengthens the mind; provides clarity and cleansing.
Green	Heals, repairs; performs all healing through the power of love.
Blue	Cools, eliminates; acts as an astringent; reduces inflammation; encourages calm and attracts spiritual guidance.
Indigo	Purifies, electrifies; provides understanding through the delivery of wisdom.
Violet	Inspires, clarifies; marries psychic and physical energies to transform negativity into positivity.
White	Awakens, perfects; ushers in spiritual energies.
Black	Empowers; erases karma; connects a being to mystical dimensions.
Silver	Reflective; deflects negativity so higher knowledge can transform a situation.
Gold	Empowering; summons the Spirit's power to effect immediate change.
Pink	Protective, loving; blends red and white to assure physical protection and spiritual results.

5: Involve Healing Streams. Concentrate on the healing statement. You can speak it aloud, chant it, or simply hold it within your heart. Then raise your hands.

Touch your pet, hold your hands in their energetic field, or simply think about your pet while your hands are raised. Now psychically picture the chosen colors and ask the Spirit to interweave these into the healing statement using healing streams of grace. You might feel these intermingled energies within or outside of your hands. Then ask the Spirit to send the entire mix of energies into the pet at the correct amplitudes and refractions. Continue this process until the energy "runs dry."

6: *Conclude.* When finished, shake your hands and ask the Spirit to release you from the healing process. Thank all concerned for what has occurred and return to your everyday life.

This exercise sets you up perfectly to deliver healing through an acupoint, the subject of the next tip.

Additional Tip

The Acupoint for Releasing Shock

The body of evidence proving the effectiveness of meridian-based therapy on pets is exponentially growing. For instance, studies show that acupuncture has successfully benefited domestic animals with relief from pain, diarrhea, spinal cord injury, Cushing's syndrome, lung function, hepatitis, and other conditions (Habacher 2006).

Why not benefit your own pet with this age-old medicine? In this section I'll show you how to employ a specific acupoint on a needy pet. It is Governing Vessel 26 (GV-26), also called the Du Mai and a revival point. GV-26 is one of several points on the Governing Vessel, a meridian that runs between the top of the forehead and the back of the spine. It manages yang, or male, energy. Stimulation of this point promotes mental alertness and recovery from shock, whether the trauma is recent or long-term. I believe that firing up this point can summon a pet's soul back into its body if a crisis has partially jettisoned it.

It's easiest to locate GV-26 on mammals and rodents, as their meridians are equivalent to a human's. All species have meridians, although the way they flow, as well as the placement of the acupoints, varies from species to species. You can learn about pet-specific meridians and points in the classic book *Traditional Chinese Veterinary Acupuncture and Moxibustion.* Showcasing fifty years of research by Professor Chuan Yu, this book illustrates the meridians of pigs, dogs, cats, rabbits, turtles, birds, ducks, chickens, rats, ferrets, hamsters, guinea pigs, horses, and other species (Yu 1995).

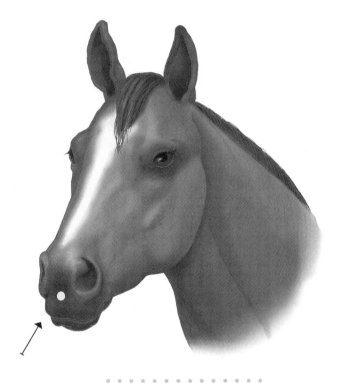

Figure 12: The Location of the Shock Acupoint

Governing Vessel 26 (GV-26), indicated by the white dot in the illustration, can be pressed to reduce stress and release shock. It is found between the nose and the upper lip in mammals and rodents and the equivalent areas in other pets.

If you want to employ GV-26, employ the entirety of the exercise "Hands-Based Healing with Color and Intention," with two main differences. In the step "Create a Healing Statement," formulate this healing statement:

I intend that the Spirit stimulate GV-26 to release my pet from shock and promote healing.

Then, in the step "Involve Healing Streams," substitute the following actions for what is written:

Concentrate on the healing statement. Say it aloud, chant it, or simply focus on it within your heart. Then locate GV-26 on your pet.

As shown on figure 12, GV-26 is found between the lip and the nose of mammals and rodents or the related area in other types of pets. For instance, in birds it is positioned above the center of the upper mandible and below the nares. You can also use the fifth chakra or auric field as a focus.

Now press the point physically or psychically in your mind, rubbing or putting pressure on it for about a minute. I suggest using your index finger, even if you are only visualizing. Ask that healing streams deliver the healing statement with the selected colors.

You can now conclude the exercise. Next, we'll learn how to soothe your pet's issues in a lovely way: music.

Toning and Music
Soothing the Pet's Soul

Human and nonhuman nations are highly affected by sound, such as tones, chants, music, and noise. In regard to pets, researcher Charles Snowdon, an animal psychologist at the University of Wisconsin-Madison, has discovered that a pet responds to species-specific music, or sounds and music uniquely composed of the pitches, tones, and tempos that suit their species. This means that we have to form sounds that relate to the pet, not ourselves, if we seek to benefit a pet.

Many species respond to noises higher or lower than those in the human range. For instance, research shows that monkeys, which are shrill creatures, calmed down when the songs were octaves higher than the sounds that soothe humans. (And if you have a pet monkey, good luck! They are very active and usually considered too wild to be suitable pets.) Cats like music that is faster in tempo than liked by humans, primarily because their heart rates are faster than ours. And, interestingly, large dogs like music that humans relate to, but small dogs, which have faster heartbeats, get jazzed by a quicker beat (Wolchover, n.d.).

A collection of studies featured on rescueanimalmp3.org showcases a sampling of the research behind this new discipline of composing music for pets (Rescue Animal MP3 Project, n.d.). I've summarized these studies for you.

First, the research establishes the fact that different components of music can change the way we think. This statement applies to human and nonhuman nations. One (human) study recorded responses to two main types of alternating chords: tritones and the perfect fifth. Researchers discovered that those listening to the triton chords thought in broader and more inclusive categories than those hearing the perfect fifths. They concluded that differing pieces of music can stimulate deeply personal but also highly specific patterns of thoughts and emotions.

The research on pets was equally revelatory. One study revealed that chicks prefer consonant rather than dissonant sounds, most likely because nature's sounds are usually consonant. And stressed dogs became calmer listening to classical music rather than heavy metal or no music, with harp music producing the same soothing effect (Rescue Animal MP3 Project, n.d.). In conclusion, the right music produces strong healing responses.

How might you formulate healing sounds for your pet? Remember to modulate your voice and tone. You can also download recordings specific to your pet; the internet features a growing body of music assisting various pet species. And the following exercise will teach you how to employ the chakra tones shared in chapter 3.

You see, chakras aren't species-specific. All pets share the same twelve chakras. Chakra tones bypass the specifics of a pet's species, whether you form the sounds aloud or internally. Try them and see!

Exercise

Sounding the Chakras into Balance

The following exercise will help you balance each pet chakra and then merge their tones into a lovely concerto. Simply follow these steps:

> **1: Prepare.** Your pet can be present or not, although sounding is often most useful if the pet is near you. Decide if you want to hum, sound, chant, or sing. All sounds can be delivered aloud or silently.

> **2: Conduct Spirit-to-Spirit.** Affirm your spirit, your pet's spirit, and the Spirit.

> **3: Tone the Chakra Spread.** One sound at a time, chant the chakra tones in the order presented below. Focus your mind on the corresponding chakra area as you proceed. If appropriate, hold a hand over the pet's related bodily area. I've written the tone with the correct spelling. In the third column, I've clued you in to the tone's pronunciation.

CHART: *Chakra Tones*

Chakra	Tone	Pronunciation
First Chakra	Lam	Lum
Second Chakra	Vam	Vum
Third Chakra	Ram	Rum
Fourth Chakra	Yam	Yum
Fifth Chakra	Ham	Hum
Sixth Chakra	Om	Aum
Seventh Chakra	Om	Aum
Eighth Chakra	Akasha	Ah-kah-sha
Ninth Chakra	Samata	Sa-ma-ta
Tenth Chakra	Ahimsa	A-him-sa
Eleventh Chakra	Seva	Say-va
Twelfth Chakra	Aham	Ah-hahm

> **5: Attune All the Chakras.** Now focus on the pet's fourth chakra and hum the yam (*yum*), requesting that the heart center attune with all other chakras through the power of love.

> **6: Close.** Conclude when you feel finished and return to your life.

Essential Oils for Pleasing and Healing Pets

Essential oils are highly concentrated reductions of plants' natural oils. They are made from plant parts, including stem and flowers, and distilled by steam or water. The remaining extraction contains the essence of the plant but also its healing properties, which can be therapeutic physically, psychologically, and behaviorally.

Essential oils have been part of the human healing protocol for centuries. As long as you use them safely, they can be a vital addition to your pet healing kit. As explained by holistic veterinarian Melissa Shelton, the key is to select and deliver oils with the species in mind (Shelton 2012).

One of my first experiences with an oil for a pet occurred at a veterinarian chiropractor. I brought in my dog Honey for an adjustment. He was so nervous that he was shaking. The first thing the chiropractor did was rub lavender oil on the top of Honey's head. After spending several minutes trying to rub off the offending smell, Honey calmed down. Lavender is quieting, and it worked. He was pliable throughout the rest of the session.

Why is it so critical to research oils before you use them? Certain oils or applications are dangerous to specific species. Essential oils are biological, and very small amounts can aid or harm a pet's system. They might contain contaminants that cause reactions or disturb an animal's sense of smell. Cats in particular are reactive or averse to many oils, mainly because cats have unusual livers and process oils differently than other animals do. For many species, the "hot" oils, like oregano and clove, should be avoided altogether, as they can burn. Neither should essential oils be put into a pet's ears or placed around the eyes, and usually they must be diluted more heavily than done for humans (Scott, n.d.).

On the other hand, properly used essential oils can be startlingly beneficial. One of my favorite studies analyzed the effects of five different types of aromatic stimulation (the control oil, lavender, chamomile, rosemary, and peppermint) on the actions of fifty-five dogs in a rescue shelter. Lavender and chamomile helped the dogs rest and relax; they also vocalized less. Rosemary and peppermint resulted in more movement and vocalization (Graham 2005).

What oils should you select for your pet and how might you apply them? I'll answer this two-part question with information credited to Dr. Stephen Blake, a well-established holistic veterinarian who employs many forms of vibrational and holistic treatments.

As shared by Dr. Blake, the following oils convey the described energies. There are many other oils available; this is merely a sampling.

CHART: *Essential Oils and Their Qualities*

Oil	Qualities
Basil	Anti-inflammatory; soothes intestines; reduces muscle spasms and mental fatigue; must be diluted with a carrier oil
Bergamot	Analgesic, natural cortisone; helps the spine
Cedar	Antibacterial; helps with dandruff, hair, and respiratory issues
Chamomile	Skin, hair care, inflamed joints; soothes
Cypress	Antimicrobial, including antiparasitic
Eucalyptus	Respiratory system, sinuses, allergies, yeast infections
Frankincense	Has helped with cancers and bolsters immune system
Juniper	Nerve stimulator, cleanser; assists with certain skin conditions
Lavender	Cuts, bruises, burns, lice; soothes and calms; a universal oil
Lemongrass	Ligaments; cleanses, purifies, and restores mental balance
Myrrh	Gum infections, skin rashes
Peppermint	Headaches, sore muscles; stimulates
Valerian	Calming, tranquilizing; for sleep and tension
Ylang Ylang	Antidepressant and calming; hypertension (Blake, n.d.)

Here are a few ideas about ways to deliver essentil oils:

Diffusion: Involves diffusing (or dispensing) the oils into the air. Because the resulting mist can be smelled, the process is called aromatherapy. The diffusion can be done passively, such as through natural evaporation, or actively, using a tool like a diffuser or spritzer bottle.

Dilution: Oils are often diluted into distilled water or into a carrier oil, such as almond oil, which can be directly delivered into food, water, or a mouth, beak, or equivalent.

Direct Application: For pets, most essential oils are diluted first into a carrier oil and then, depending on the species, dabbed on the fur, paws, or comparable part of the body. Raindrop Therapy involves applying oils to various parts of the body through targeted massage and touch. This process can alleviate emotional as well as physical and structural issues and is frequently used with chiropractic and acupuncture modalities.

Environmental Application: Depending on the species, drops or atomized solutions can be delivered into or next to a pet's environment, such as a cage, stable, or bedding.

Given the energetic relationship between us and our pets, we can also use an oil on ourselves and ask for healing streams to send the oil's energy to the pet. Put the oil on yourself, conduct Spirit-to-Spirit, and ask that healing streams carry the subtle frequencies of the oil to your pet, dispensing them wherever they would be useful.

As stated, you must be pet-specific in the selection and application of oil. I recommend seeking professional advice or using Dr. Melissa Shelton's book, *The Animal Desk Reference: Essential Oils for Animals.* Her advice is quite detailed. For instance, when treating a bird for arthritis, you'll choose between several helpful oils, including balsam fir, copaiba, frankincense, lavender, lemon, myrrh, peppermint, and more. One of Shelton's recommended treatments involves mixing 10 drops of frankincense and 5 drops of copaiba in 4 ounces of distilled water. This blend is then mixed and directly misted on the bird one to two times a day (Shelton 2012, 255).

There is yet another natural essence that can be truly helpful. It is made from flowers.

Flower Essences
The Blooms of Life

Flower essences are tinctures made from small amounts of wildflowers. The original creator of flower essences was Dr. Edward Bach, who invented his flower formulas between 1920 and 1930. Safe for humans and pets, the original thirty-eight formulas enhance or restore balance between the mind, body, and soul, also relieving a pet's disturbing emotions, such as fear and worry. These remedies are perfect for helping your pets with their psychological issues.

Most of the remedies contain alcohol, however, which is not healthy for certain types of pets, especially birds and smaller animals. You can dilute the amount of essence given to small creatures by mixing the remedy in a bottle or looking for alcohol-free remedies; there are a few sold on various Bach remedy websites. As there isn't any information about using Bach Flower essences with reptiles, amphibians, and arthropods, I'd recommend working with a pet naturopath or holistic veterinarian if interested.

To dose and deliver Bach Flower remedies, first visit bachflowerpets.com to learn more about the remedies and how to dose them for pets. In general, remedies come ready to go in bottles with a dropper. You can add drops of a selected essence to a water dish or food. You can also rub the dosage on their gums, place it under the tongue, or drop the remedy into a beak. Remedies can also be dabbed on paw pads or its equivalent body part, patted behind an ear, or mixed into a misting bottle. The resulting mist can be sprayed over an animal or in a habitat. If you want to be extra cautious, spray *near* a habitat. If you share an issue with your pet, take the remedy yourself and ask that healing streams transfer the essence's frequency from you to your pet.

Know that there are other types of essential remedies, made of everything from flowers to trees, but the original essences were made by Bach. Following is a chart outlining the pet remedies actually recommended on the Bach website. I've added my sense of which chakra relates to which remedy as well. If you can't select a remedy based on symptoms, you can then pick one based on a causal chakra.

CHART: *Bach Flower Essences by Chakra*

Chakra	Symptoms	Bach Remedy	Outcome
First	Stressful situations; fear of noises and change; anything causing insecurity	Rescue Remedy, a universal remedy dealing with shock, pain, and acute challenges	Immediate calming
Second	Unfriendliness and standoffish attitudes	Water Violet	Sociability and compassion
Third	Lack of self-confidence; avoidance of situations requiring performance	Larch	Increased self-esteem and confidence
Fourth	Neediness; abandonment issues; manipulates for love	Chicory	Unselfish and loving approach to relationships
Fifth	Makes angry noises; jealousy and aggressiveness	Holly	More compassion and calm; willingness to share
Sixth	Lack of direction or purpose	Wild Oat	Restoration of ambition and purpose
Seventh	Out of control physicality; frenzied motion; prefers to be alone	Impatiens	Increased patience and wisdom; willingness to connect
Eighth	Has been abused or acts abused; was mistreated in the past; trauma can be carried in karmically	Star of Bethlehem	Neutralization of shock and trauma, often through processing of karma
Ninth	Dreaminess; sleepiness; no interest in surrounding world	Clematis	Enjoyment of life; increased interaction
Tenth	Stuck in the past; could also be stuck in ancestors' pasts or early childhood; loss of home or owner	Honeysuckle	Awareness of the present; appreciation of surroundings; adaptation to new environment
Eleventh	Authoritative and domineering	Vine	Shift into leadership; release of need to dominate
Twelfth	Obsessiveness. I believe that all obsessive qualities represent lack of self-acceptance and prevent the unique twelfth chakra from activating.	Crab Apple	Improved sense of clarity; acceptance of imperfections and the entire self. Unique qualities can then be activated.

It's now time to learn about yet another vibrational remedy, one often considered as much a medicine as many found in the allopathic medical bag.

Homeopathy
Hope and Healing

Homeopathy is a healing approach founded in the late 1700s in Germany. It differs philosophically from allopathic medicine in that symptoms of an illness or imbalance are considered a normal response to an emotional, physical, or environmental challenge. The vibrations of the malady can therefore be seen to enhance the body's regular healing processes.

Typically, homeopathic practitioners employ liquid tinctures or small pills called "remedies" that stimulate a physical, psychological, and spiritual response. Remedies are made from natural substances, including plants, minerals, chemicals, spiders, and insects.

Homeopathy can be prescribed for dogs, cats, horses, and other mammals and rodents, and to a lesser extent for fish, birds, and reptiles, including snakes, lizards, turtles, and iguanas. In fact, research suggests that nearly any nonhuman being can be treated with homeopathy. Interestingly, according to the British Homeopathic Association, dosage for a natural being is the same as for a human (British Homeopathic Association, n.d.).

Following are a few homeopathic pet remedies. I heartily recommend that you consider using an expert to select remedies if you have any doubts or confusion. Homeopathy is a real medicine, and its usage depends on choosing the correct treatment but also dosage and frequency.

Keeping this in mind, how might you deliver homeopathy to a pet? Mammals and rodents can be treated directly with a tincture put in a food or water bowl. A bird's treatment is usually delivered under the beak or in the water. For reptiles and amphibians, the remedy can be dissolved or dropped into a water source, and fish are best treated by medicating the water they swim in. For other types of beings, I'd consult a professional or use healing streams to subtly bring the energy into the pet. You can simply hold the remedy and ask that healing streams convey it energetically to the pet.

Following is a short list of beneficial homeopathic remedies. You'll notice that the same condition, such as anxiety, is treated with different remedies, depending on symptoms. The complexity of arriving at a treatment again underscores my point. Consult a professional if you have any questions.

CHART: *Homeopathic Remedies for Pets*

Symptom	Remedy
Anxiety with abject fear	Gelsemium
Anxiety with anguish	Ars
Anxiety when first felt	Aconite
Anxiety with overstimulation	Lycopodium
Anxiety in reaction to thunderstorms and loud noises	Phos
Back injuries, all	Arnica
Back injuries with violent pain	Bell
Bites from other pets	Aconite, Arnica
Bone injuries	Arnica, Aconite
Burns and scalds	Aconite
Colic with a swollen, tender abdomen	Bell
Cystitis with straining and blood	Canth
Cystitis with full blockage	Uva ursi
Ear infections	Hepar
Food poisoning	Arsenicum
Hives with itchy skin and clingy behavior	Nat mur
Hives with puffy and red skin	Apis
Hives with small red bumps and intense itching	Rhus tox
Injuries to tail, paws, claws, or toes	Hypher
Pain	Aconite
Puncture wounds and insect bites	Ledum
Orphaned	Aconite or Calc phos
Shock	Aconite
Shyness	Pulsatilla
Toxicity or poisoning	Nux-vomica
Trauma	Arnica, often given after aconite
Travel sickness when moving, such as in a car	Cocc
Travel sickness caused by fear in advance of travel	Gels

(Whistler Veterinarian Clinic, n.d.; Day 2002; Walker, n.d., 21, 32, 41, 51, 57, 63, 79, 106, 121–122, 144, 147).

As we round the corner of this chapter, we find ourselves back at our beginning: stones.

Stone Therapy for Pets

We established the benefit of stone therapy in the beginning of this chapter. Stone therapy includes the use of crystals but also regular rocks, including river and volcanic stones. If you decide to employ stone therapy with your pet—and I really hope you do—there are three main considerations. The first is how to use a stone with a pet. I mean, pets don't exactly have pockets in which to carry stones. The second involves figuring out which stone to use. The third is attuning the stone so it meets your pet's needs. I'll cover all three issues in this section and then provide you an exercise for programming a stone for your pet's needs.

As for introducing a stone (or number of stones) into your pet's life, you can use the following methods:

- Setting the stone in a pet's bedding or cage, stall, tank, or other habitat.

- Embedding the stone in a collar, saddle, or leash.

- Putting the stone in a drinking bowl, water holder, or tank, or spraying it as an atomizer. Because some stones are toxic, use the process described after this list to create any liquid stone medicines.

- Placing the stone around the habitat, perhaps in an ornamental fashion.

- Carrying around the stone yourself, especially when around the pet.

- Holding the stone when using the exercises in the prior chapters to help perform pet communication or empower healing streams.

- Certain stones are always toxic if ingested by pets or people, including galena, torbernite, and cinnabar. Yet others are harmful to specific types of pets. Because of this, it's important to use the formula I'm going to share if you want to deliver stone magic in liquid form, such as through a tincture or an atomizer spray. Basically, you'll need a stone or stones, a glass, distilled water, and a pitcher. You'll want to be able to put the glass inside of the pitcher, as you'll basically be making your stone solution with water in the glass and using healing streams to send the subtle energy of the solution into the water held within the pitcher.

- Start with your glass. Fill it with distilled water. Take a clean stone and plop it into the glass. If using multiple stones, the ratio of stones to water is one-third to two-thirds. Conduct Spirit-to-Spirit and ask the Spirit to send healing streams into the water; simultaneously focus on an intention. Your focus can be as simple as this: "Clear and activate this stone for its highest use." It can also be specific: "Vitalize this water to heal my pet of emotional stress."

- Now add some distilled water to the pitcher and place the glass in it. Do not let the fluids mix. Use Spirit-to-Spirit and ask that the healing streams in the smaller glass deliver the stone's properties and the established intention into the water in the surrounding pitcher. Then leave the entire contraption as-is for about twelve hours. You can set it in moonlight or sunlight for an extra boost. When finished, remove the glass. You'll use the water within the pitcher as your "medicine." Pour it into a dispensing bottle for use as a tincture or atomizer.

How do you know which stone to employ? There are thousands of different stones, and each resonates with a different vibration. You'll basically want to compose an intention and select a stone that matches the pet's need. Also figure out if you want to perform healing, manifesting, or both. As shared previously, healing is the release of unnecessary or unhealthy energies. Manifesting is the attraction of a desirable energy. Sometimes you want to accomplish both, in which case you'll need to select a stone for each objective.

The following chart will help you select the best stone for a pet. These stones are nontoxic for pets. Nonetheless, if creating a liquid, use the formula that I just provided. Also make sure that the pet can't swallow the stone and that if the stone is to be placed near a pet, its edges are blunt.

CHART: *Stones by Chakras and Influences*

Stone	Chakra/s	Influences
Amber	Third, Tenth	Absorbs negative energy; awakens the bond with nature; opens hidden ancestral wisdom; regulates eccentricities; assures altruism. (Use to substitute ancient wisdom for anxiety and mental dysfunction.)
Amethyst	Sixth	Activates clairvoyance and psychic insights; deflects negativity. (Employ when releasing attachments and entities.)
Citrine	Third	Assures mental clarity; improves memory; restores confidence; heals digestion. (Use to dissolve emotions.)
Coral	Second	Encourages activity, courage, forcefulness, and emotional balance. (Excellent remedy to create joy in reptiles, amphibians, and fish.)
Diamond	Seventh, Eighth, Ninth, Tenth, Eleventh	Amplifies strengths and weaknesses; clears blocks; activates chakra's spiritual power. (Use to diagnose karma and activate dharma.)
Emerald	Fourth	Increases confidence, abundance, peacefulness, and fidelity. (Perfect stone for improving relationships.)
Fluorite	All	Delivers cleansing and protection. (There are many colors of fluorite. Select the hue matching the chakra and auric field needing cleansing and fortification.)
Limestone	Tenth	Enables grounding and stability. (Use to bolster energetic boundaries and create a practical outcome.)
Moldavite	Eighth	Awakens memories of past lives; makes interdimensional connections. (Employ the stone to connect to beings from other planes, planets, and time periods.)
Pearl	Seventh, Ninth	Downloads higher wisdom into the pet; harmonizes what is disharmonious; attunes to the cycles of nature. (Use to help a pet transcend circumstances.)
River Rock	Second, Fourth	Represents energies of water, increasing intuition and flow of feelings. (Use to heal any emotional disorder.)
Ruby	First	Creates physical oneness with the Spirit; protects from evil; helps release the wounded self from shock. (Employ whenever the Spirit's power is needed.)

Stone	Chakra/s	Influences
Sapphire, Blue	Fifth	Heals perfectionist tendencies; relieves misery; assures higher communication. (Can clear communication disorders, including those involving another pet, human, or spiritual guide.)
Turquoise	Sixth	Links to higher spiritual guidance and loving sources of wisdom; accesses truths from any culture and age. (Employ to release old hurts and bring in wisdom of the ages.)
Quartz, Pink	All	Assures feelings of love, peacefulness, and forgiveness. (Can be used for any purpose, as love is the highest of powers.)
Quartz, White	All	Delivers clarity; cleanses and purifies. (Brings the Spirit or spiritual guides into any situation.)
Volcanic Rock	First, Tenth	Represents fire energy; purifies, cleanses, renews. (Use to burn away physical and psychic toxicity and develop wisdom.)

Exercise

Easy Stone Programming

Want to quickly and easily program a stone for a higher intention? Refer to the listing just provided and take the following steps.

> 1: *Prepare.* Select a stone based on your purpose. If unclear, use the pet communication techniques taught in chapter 5 to specifically check out a stone with your pet. Also trust your body. If a stone feels right for your pet, it is. If none of the described stones seem right, there are hundreds of websites providing information about other stones. Be clear about which chakra/s you will be interacting with.

> 2: *Conduct Spirit-to-Spirit.* Affirm your spirit, your pet's spirit, and the Spirit.

> 3: *Set Your Intention.* Create an intention appropriate for your pet. The statement should be positive in nature, such as, "This stone is assisting my pet with releasing the emotions resulting from being abandoned."

4: Ask for Healing Streams. Focusing on the intention, request that the Spirit send healing streams into the stone. The streams will load the intention into the stone. When you use this stone on your pet, the healing streams will directly enter the pet—specifically into the chakra/s that need transformation, thus supporting the accomplishment of the intention. Decide how else to deliver the stone's newfound energy to your pet, selecting from the processes offered in beginning of page 187's section "Stone Therapy for Pets."

If you want to select a stone to use while performing some of the exercises in this book, I'll help you do that next.

Additional Tip

Applying Stones to Various Exercises

In chapter 6 you learned a number of exercises, each devoted to helping your pet with specific concerns. Following are a few ideas about which stones to use when employing these exercises. You can use any process desired to interact with the stone, but the easiest is to simply hold it.

Pinpointing Your Starting Spot—The Beginning of the Healing: White quartz will help clear preconceptions that might muddle your assessment.

Releasing Karmic Patterns: Moldavite will greatly bolster your ability to perceive a pet's past lives and related patterns, no matter the universe the pet once dwelled in. A diamond will uncover the karmic weaknesses of a pet and illuminate the strengths gained from a challenging experience.

Activating Dharmic Truths: A diamond will clarify any vital dharmic qualities. A pearl can open the inner wheel of a chakra and distribute the truth held within it throughout the pet's system.

Clearing Cords and Holds: Use a stone specific to the chakra infected by an attachment. If the attachment is life threatening, use a ruby. If you need a general cleansing after an attachment release, employ fluorite. Amethyst will help you deflect the dark energies involved

in the attachment and figure out the message or wisdom your pet
needs to receive to move on.

Clearing the Trauma Pathway: Select a stone specific to a chakra or
bodily site. Also consider the following: blue sapphire for hearing
the traumatized self; amber to cleanse the pathway with needed
subtle elements; amethyst to clear out cords and holds and erect
better energetic boundaries; ruby to blast out negative energies
and reestablish a connection with the Spirit; citrine or coral to
rescue a wounded pet from the shock bubble; diamond to clear
blocks and assess the affects of a trauma; moldavite to uncover
the karmic causes for a trauma; fluorite to promote cleansing of
entrance and exit wounds, stuck energies, and the overall pathway;
pearl and turquoise to introduce the once-shocked self to new and
higher truths; emerald to establish loving relationships after a subtle
clearing; and pink or white quartz to encourage clarity and love.

Separating Emotions: Use blue sapphire to enhance communication
with a pet's soul or wounded self; citrine or coral to perform
emotional analysis and healing; pearl, emerald, or diamond to
enable proper relationships; and turquoise to help the pet access
higher truths. Pink and white quartz can always be used for
cleansing purposes.

Transforming Microbes: Amber can help you intuitively assess which
microbes are affecting a pet. It can also link your pet to energies
in nature or the cosmos that can provide clearing. Ruby assists
with detaching viruses from an external force. Citrine and coral
support a pet in feeling the feelings trapped in bacteria. Amethyst
can separate a pet from parasitic energies and help it establish a
bond with the Spirit, and fluorite will assist a pet with releasing the
energies held within yeast, molds, and fungi.

Now that you've explored the fantastic world of vibrational medicines, it's time
to lift our discussion to another level, one definitely more supernatural in that
it relates to death, dying, and the afterlife—to happy endings.

Chapter Eight
Of Dying, Death, and the Afterlife

...love knows not its own depth
until the hour of separation.

Kahlil Gibran

There is nothing more difficult than the death of a pet, except maybe the actual dying process. Our heart breaks when our beloved friend is suffering. It breaks again when the pet dies and we must surrender to our loss. Because of this, it's all the more important to understand the energetic and spiritual nature of a pet's death and dying process. This knowledge is imperative to supporting our pet and ourselves through—and beyond—this most difficult of times.

In this chapter we'll explore issues related to all stages of the transitional process, which are dying, death, and the afterlife, covering what occurs energetically in each phase. After exploring the energetics of these stages, I'll zero in on particulars related to each, such as the reasons that a pet might die and the various forms of dying. I'll also provide an exercise you can use if you're questioning the timing of your pet's demise.

I'll then describe what happens on the soul level after a pet's death, providing an exercise you can use to both release your pet and also communicate with them once they have passed. In the end, you'll see that endings aren't really endings but new beginnings.

When It's Time to Leave

Throughout this book, I've talked frequently about my dog Honey, the golden retriever. I've probably confused you, unless you've read about Honey in a couple of my other books, as Honey has a complicated history. The Honey that currently resides with me is actually Honey III. He has been alive at least twice before.

The first Honey lived with my son Gabe's father decades ago. The first Honey was a male golden retriever. To honor that history, despite being divorced from Gabe's father, I bought a male golden retriever puppy for my son. Of course we named it Honey. I knew enough stories about Honey I to quickly surmise that Honey I and Honey II were the same soul.

For instance, Honey I used to steal food from the neighbors; in fact, he once devoured a neighbor's unguarded picnic meal. He loved to eat so much he would jog over to a local Italian restaurant every morning for free meatballs. Honey II displayed the same characteristic.

One time, a huge truck pulled up to my house. A man rang my bell and asked if I owned a golden retriever. Puzzled, I said yes. The man led me to his truck. There sat Honey II in the passenger seat, grinning. Apparently, Honey II had snuck out of my backyard and jumped into the workers' open truck, thereby consuming their lunches. My neighbors instantly knew who had eaten the food; Honey II had quite the reputation.

Honey II was my son's best friend. They slept together. They ate alongside of each other. At every show-and-tell in elementary school, Gabe shared pictures of Honey II. But when Honey II was seven years old, he was stricken with a throat disease. I brought him to a critical care hospital, but after two days I had to put him down.

Afterward, I tried to figure out the reason for Honey II's sudden demise. I received no intuitive guidance until a few weeks after Honey II's death. I was at the movies and I heard a voice say, "I left to save Gabe."

I still have no idea what calamity might have befallen my son, but I know that Honey II and my son were karmically interconnected through Gabe's father's side of the family. Obviously, there was also a dharmic signature that bonded Gabe and Honey. Honey II had taken a blow for my son. That type of unconditional love and sacrifice is rare.

We moved on. About three years later, I was awakened by a voice: "I'm coming back!" I groaned. Honey II had been incredibly busy and wild.

That same morning my son came into my room. He'd found a male golden retriever puppy on the internet and insisted that we buy it. The puppy's name was Tank, and he lived in Pennsylvania. The inevitable happened, despite my resistance; I was forced into getting Honey III. The universe conspired against me. Everywhere my son and I went for days after, we saw tanks: Sherman tanks, toilet tanks, GI Joe tanks. Honey, the nectar, was delivered to the house. I hadn't ordered it. I had no choice but to buy Tank after a discussion with my therapist.

My therapist worked in a no-pet building. I had been discussing the quandary of purchasing Tank or not during the session. My final words on the matter, as I was stepping out of her office, were these: "I just need one more sign before I pull the plug." What happened? A dog rushed up to me in the hallway, holding a leash in its mouth. I went home and bought Tank.

That wasn't the end of the story, karmic or dharmic.

About a week after Honey III moved in, Lucky, my yellow Labrador, bit him in the nose. I rushed Honey III to the same emergency veterinarian hospital I had brought Honey II during his demise. Honey III was injured in the same bodily area that had caused Honey II's death. However, he underwent the surgery he hadn't qualified for as Honey II and lived. Now that his karma is complete, he's happily ensconced in our family. Only this time, he's even more oral. He absolutely never stops eating or talking.

I've hinted at his proclivities for squeaky toys, but there is more to the story. When I'm running the dogs in a fenced-in park every morning, Honey spends the entire time jogging about with a squeaky toy. If a person is unlucky enough to be in the park at dawn, he follows them around, squeaking at them. He's also known as the neighborhood street cleaner. A walk down the street will find him consuming everything from dropped French fries to dead mice.

Honey (every version of him) clearly demonstrates the many cycles of a pet soul, including birth, life, dying, death, the afterlife, and, potentially, a rebirth. Karma, dharma, and love are interwoven in all stages of a pet's process, and so are energetics. In fact, if you want to fully support your pet through all cycles of life and death, it's key to understanding the energetics of these matters, the subject of the next section.

The Energetics of Death and Dying

From Sea to Shining Sea

As shared, death and dying are merely two stages of a continual process that also includes birth, life, dying, death, the afterlife, and perhaps another rebirth. I perceive every one of these stages as comparable to the waves rolling at a beach: the same water—or soul—returning over and over to the surface.

As discussed in previous chapters, a pet's spirit and soul are integral to preparing the pet for the journey ahead. Both interact with specific chakras, many of which are activated during preconception. Through the eighth chakra, the soul uploads selected karmic lessons onto the outer wheel of every chakra. Meanwhile, the pet's spirit deposits spiritual qualities and dharmic goals into the inner wheel of each chakra. During conception, the karmic and dharmic attributes are then meshed through the pet's tenth chakra, which in turn encodes the genetic and epigenetic material. Additional programs, including familial, are also affixed in the outer wheel of each chakra, and finally the tiny embryo is ready to go.

A pet's soul doesn't actually enter its body until the fertilized egg starts to grow, at which time the soul anchors in the first chakra. While the ethereal energy of the soul is distributed like a vapor throughout the subtle and physical energetic systems, the substance of the soul is affixed in the body one chakra at a time. As the pet ages, the soul ascends the chakra ladder, activating the chakras' various stages of development. Finally, the pet's full energetic signature is embodied—and it is time to leave. Well, that's what happens if everything stays on track.

If a pet exits at a mature stage of development, the dying process is most likely quite peaceful, meaning it will be more dharmic and less karmic. It will also tend to exit through either the seventh, eleventh, or twelfth chakra.

As explained in chapters 3 and 4, the soul ascends into the seventh chakra during late maturity. The soul that dies or exits at this time makes its way straight into one of the planes of light or spiritual realms I'll describe later in this chapter. If a soul doesn't leave at this point, it jumps up the chakra ladder into the eleventh chakra, entering a stage that is quite amenable to death. At this point, the pet might exhibit supernatural abilities or cause the same in the environment. Upon death, the soul can exit through this chakra, which provides a tranquil and illuminating death, but it can also depart through the unique twelfth chakra. If this occurs, the soul achieves a sort of fulfillment and is free to be its true self.

All pets have the same chance of transcending through the chakras in the way I just described, no matter how long they live. House ants live about three years, but they can still evolve through all chakras during that time. Even if an ant's life is truncated, the soul can progress through all remaining chakra stages in a moment, hour, or day, quickly assimilating the lessons involved in each chakra stage. In fact, any soul can do this. Then again, some souls hardly get out of the gate, despite living a relatively long life. Trauma can cause the soul to become stuck in a lower chakra, and there it remains.

Even when a soul is stuck, the soul can hope for a transcendent exodus. As mentioned, a soul can soar through the chakras in a split second. There are also parts of a pet's soul that don't become embodied in every lifetime. The more advanced aspects can leap into the body at any stage of the dying process and help the soul ascend to the light when dying. But, as implied, challenging circumstances can negatively affect the dying soul.

One particularly difficult situation is a sudden death. Especially when traumatic, the shock can cause the pet's soul to jettison out of the damaged chakra. Unready for death, the soul might become confused or muddled. As we'll discuss further in this chapter, the soul might wander the earth plane for a while or not even know that it is dead. In these cases, the dead soul might need help to be released from the earthly realm. Later in this chapter you'll be taught an exercise, "Releasing Your Pet with Love," to assist with these and other challenging situations.

As you can surmise, there are a lot of complications involved in death and dying. The human who loves their pet can make a significant difference in these processes by better understanding the energetic complexities. We'll start by discussing the first of the stages, which is the dying process.

Dying

The First Stage of a Pet's Passing

What actually occurs spiritually and energetically when a pet is dying? The answer depends on the differing reasons a pet dies, as well as how it dies. As I explore these factors, I'll include a few recommendations about how to help your pet and its loved ones, including yourself, through the various possibilities.

The Four Reasons a Pet Dies

There are four main reasons that a pet dies. These are karmic, dharmic, inopportune, and chaotic. Each reason is marked by different signs and should be supported in different ways, as I'll explain.

Karmic Dying

Karmic deaths enable a pet to work through a historically difficult issue. Frequently, a karmic death is a repeat of a prior death. The underlying spiritual reason for repeating a previous death is to unearth love. For instance, I have a client whose horse, Moxie, died from an acute injury. Ben came to see me while Moxie was dying.

Together, Ben and I connected to Moxie's soul. Moxie showed both of us psychically that he and Ben had been through this type of event in a previous lifetime. Ben had been a soldier in the Civil War and Moxie had been his horse. They became separated in the battle and Moxie had died from a gunshot wound, scared and alone. The sense was that this time, Ben needed to be at Moxie's side so that Moxie could know himself as loved. Ben did this. He returned after Moxie's death and said that he had never felt so connected to another living being as he had the dying Moxie. He believed the same was true for Moxie. The karmic teaching—the lesson that love is eternal—was gifted to both Ben and Moxie's souls.

Sometimes the dying pet has taken on a loved one's karma. This was the case with Honey II, who died so that something negative didn't happen to my son. Other times the pet is caught in a repetitive loop it can't get out of; for instance, it has always suffered a traumatic death. Whatever the karma, the key characteristics of a karmic dying process include the sense of repetition, the feeling that the ending can't be changed, and the perception that though love can't alter the outcome, it can make the process better. When assisting the karmically passing pet, see if you can attune to the issues the soul is working through. Use your pet communication tools to relate directly to the pet's soul. Ask if there is a past life to understand or a current life trauma to clear. If you can, relate the karma to a chakra and release the trauma using the skills taught already in this book.

Dharmic Dying

Sometimes a pet dies and the process is so loving, or creates so many loving after-effects, that you know the pet's passing is dharmic or blessed. For instance, I worked with a client whose elderly cat underwent a six-month dying process. At the end, the cat easily passed from the seventh to the eleventh and then twelfth chakra stage of development. How do I know? I'll share two stories.

Kitty's human companion, Granny, had lived alone on her farm for years. Because Kitty was dying, Granny's relatives started visiting Kitty. After Kitty died, one of Granny's daughters set up a visitation schedule so Granny would never be alone. Kitty the cat earned five stars, living out her energetic signature of assuring community and caring. But that wasn't the last that Granny nor her relatives saw of—or heard from—Kitty.

After Kitty died, she appeared in two forms, one as a cat, another as a winged being. Whenever Granny felt really lonely, Kitty would appear as a cat made of white vapor. As such, she padded around the house and purred; sometimes she slept with Granny. Other times, however, Kitty looked like a huge winged creature and would issue warnings to Granny to deliver to a loved one. Granny knew that it was Kitty because of the being's basic nature, which Granny said "was Kitty-like." Once, Granny called her grandson and told him that Kitty had issued a warning about a semi truck. "When your grandson sees a semi truck where it isn't supposed to be, tell him to pull off the road," the creature had insisted. Later that day, the grandson saw a semi on a side road while driving. He pulled to the side just before the semi blew a tire and teetered around violently. Had he not heeded Kitty's warning, the grandson would have been hurt. My theory is that Kitty's dharmic self had even further evolved since death, perhaps because she existed through her twelfth chakra, and she could now be her fullest and uniquely gifted self.

Dharmic dying processes can leave us sad and scared, but they also evoke compassion and love. They might bring nonhuman or human beings together and reveal the love hidden within a relationship. To support a pet in this process, figure out the gift or wisdom the pet is bestowing. You can assess the pet's energetic signature to gain clues. Make sure the pet is only surrounded by caring people or natural beings at the end; this isn't the time to cause the pet to trigger old—or form new—issues.

Inopportune Dying

Many people wonder if a pet's death or dying process is preordained. Sometimes it is. Most souls (human and nonhuman) preselect several exit points before birth.

When a pet departs during a preordained point, the event might be painful or shocking, but it seems destined. When pets leave at non-arranged times, the process feels "off." For instance, I worked with a young client who startled her pet bunny so much that it hopped out of the house, only to be run over by a car. The girl didn't think that was supposed to happen.

Intuitively, I sensed that the bunny had departed before its destined time. I knew, however, that a rabbit's species code includes being easily scared. I helped the girl understand that through this event, the bunny had learned a lesson it could carry into another life. The girl could transform the tragedy by embracing the same lesson—something like "think before acting." Years later, the girl came to see me again. Reflecting upon the death of her bunny, she said that the event had taught her the importance of pausing before reacting and that, in general, she was less anxious than she used to be.

If a pet's exit seems inopportune, determine what lesson can be gleaned from the experience. This statement can apply to the pet's soul, other living pets, and involved humans. If needed, use your pet communication skills to talk with the departed pet soul and encourage it to embrace the related lesson. There are simply events beyond anyone's control, not only during life but also in relationship to death.

Chaotic Dying

There are death processes that seem wrong at every level. Some deaths occur because the world is chaotic, full of dark forces that feed the chaos. As an example, I had a client whose pet chicken died overnight. My client had spied a shadow creeping around her bedroom earlier in the night and was sure that the entity had killed her chicken. We received confirmation of this conclusion during our intuitive session.

The dark force seemed to be a malevolent "passerby" that didn't approve of joy. Therefore, the entity frightened her chicken to death so that its human companion would be unhappy. We released the entity from the chicken's soul and determined that the client needed to embrace her right to be joyful.

If you suspect that interference is causing a pet's dying process, use the pet communication skills obtained in chapter 5 to obtain input from your pet or its spiritual guide/s. Use healing streams to surround the darkness in a bubble of grace and to send it away. Check for and release cords or holds, and if the pet is in an early stage of chakra development, ask the Spirit to mature it more quickly. This way, if the pet does die, its soul will pass more peacefully.

Sooner or later, of course, every pet will die. Consider the various types of death and what each might indicate about your pet's soul and yourself.

Types of Dying

There are several ways that a pet might die. Let's look at what might be happening in the energetic realms when any of the following occur.

Sudden Deaths

The sudden death of a pet is shocking. An instant death might happen because of karma but also because the death might constitute a "dharmic gift" from the Spirit, such as occurs through a pain-free passing. The more sudden the death, the more support the remaining pets or humans need.

To help the humans, create a board of pet pictures or scrapbook, conduct a funeral or life celebration, or share memories aloud. Watch nonhuman members of a household for signs of shock, such as over- or under-sleeping, over- or under-eating, or a loss of interest in normal activities. Vibrational medicines, described in the last chapter, can greatly assist grieving pets. Also talk aloud or intuitively to your living pets about the missing pet, and use pet communication to ask the deceased pet soul to intuitively connect with its still-alive human and nonhuman loved ones, if appropriate.

In the case of a sudden death, a pet's soul might not know it's dead. If you hear pet sounds or get other indications that the pet is a ghost, use the exercise "Releasing Your Pet with Love" found on page 207 to guide your pet to the other side. Also use your knowledge of trauma healing to assist the pet's soul.

Quick Deaths

Quick deaths are different than sudden deaths in that a warning proceeds the event. Maybe your pet was diagnosed with a fast-moving cancer or organ failure. Maybe it was hit by a car but remains alive for a while. Why might a pet die quickly? Sometimes the pet's soul has an upcoming assignment, such as a new life to get to. A quick death might also spare the pet unnecessary pain. Maybe the pet's soul habitually departs quickly. If you've time, make sure the pet is comfortable and give humans and nonhumans time to say goodbye. Let other humans share their appreciation for the dying pet. Also ask the Spirit to guide the pet's soul into the seventh, eleventh, or twelfth chakra and establish healing streams to guide the soul onward.

Slow Deaths

Drawn-out deaths can be challenging, although they provide time for making peace with the inevitable. However, the long process can cause all parties to become tired, irritable, and emotional.

If the pet isn't in pain, keep it comfortable and involved in as many normal activities as possible. Use your pet communication skills to uncover any trauma or memories that need to come to light. You can also use Spirit-to-Spirit and healing streams to guide the pet's soul into a higher chakra before it dies. If the pet is in pain, read the next section.

Painful Deaths

There is nothing harder than watching a pet in pain. Consider using prescription medications and euthanizing when it feels like the correct time. A veterinarian will guide you through both steps. On the subtle level, use the trauma-clearing techniques you've learned in this book to uncover karmic or emotional memories. Physical pain is often increased by inflammatory and stuck emotions, as well as others' energies. Also send healing streams through the pet's first chakra, which governs life and death issues. This activity might quicken the death and also decrease the pain. I strongly suggest you employ vibrational medicines as well.

Peaceful Deaths

The apex of a pet's life is a peaceful death, whether it is quick or slow. Basically, a peaceful pet death occurs when its soul leaves through the higher chakras and the pet has fully embodied its personal energetic signature. At this point, the pet often emanates a spiritual energy that can be intuitively felt or seen. Most likely, this energy is psychically seen as white, rose, or gold. You might also sense the presence of spiritual guides around the pet, including pets that have already passed over. You can increase the possibility of a peaceful death by calling upon the pet's guides through prayers or by using Spirit-to-Spirit.

What if you sense that you can reverse the dying process? I have a friend whose dog was diagnosed with fourth stage cancer. The prognosis didn't feel right to her. She prayed about it, got treatment for the dog, and it lived another five years. You can use the following exercise to check for this possibility.

Exercise

Helping Your Pet Stay

What if you have a sense that your pet doesn't want or need to die yet? This simple exercise will align your pet's soul and body with the Spirit to create the highest outcome.

> 1: **Prepare.** Breathe deeply and relax. You can be in your pet's presence or not. If you want, hold a stone chosen from page 187's section "Stone Therapy for Pets."
>
> 2: **Conduct Spirit-to-Spirit.** Affirm your spirit, your pet's spirit, and its helping spirits. Then turn this process over to the Spirit, whose power is greater than any held by death.
>
> 3: **Gain Knowledge.** Ask the Spirit to reveal any necessary information about your pet's circumstances. You can ask direct questions, such as, "Is my pet supposed to survive this challenge?"
>
> You can also ask the Spirit to direct-connect you with your pet's soul. Ask the soul, "Do you want to survive or not?" If it

says yes, ask for more information. Questions can include "For what reason do you seek more time?" and "How can I best support you in recovering?"

Now return to the Spirit. If both the pet's spirit and the Spirit think that the pet's life could be extended, ask more questions about supporting the pet. You can also request a list of recommended practitioners and treatments, both allopathic and holistic.

4: Request Further Assistance. Before concluding, ask the Spirit to continue to guide you toward surrendering your pet to death or supporting it in living longer.

5: Conclude. Thank the Spirit and decide to remain open for additional insights.

After Death
The Soul's Process

When the inevitable occurs, the pet's soul departs the body. Then what happens?

Recall that while alive, the pet's soul ideally travels up the chakra ladder. During the final stages of the dying process, the soul prepares to exit. If it's mature, it leaves through the seventh, eleventh, or twelfth chakra. It can also jettison from the body through any other chakra. It is more apt to do this if the death is sudden or injurious, in which case it might depart through the damaged chakra. No matter what, at the moment of death the soul gathers the memories, feelings, and beliefs related to the just-experienced lifetime into its etheric field, the densest energetic field surrounding it. In the twelve-chakra system, this field equates with the tenth auric field. Thus the soul brings with it the awareness of the karmic issues processed and those still undone. And hopefully, it ascends with lovely dharmic achievements.

Just before death, many pet souls are visited by a "welcoming committee" of at least two spiritual beings, which grant them the psychological, spiritual, and physical assistance they need to depart in a loving way. This group can include deceased loved ones, spiritual guides, and the Spirit.

After death, the pet's soul can travel along any number of ethereal avenues. It might remain anchored in the physical world, at least for a while. This usually happens if a cord exists between a pet's soul, another pet, or a human companion; if the death was shocking; or if the pet is too traumatized to leave. As well, the soul might not realize it's dead, or it might want to continue taking care of its family. Technically, any pet soul that remains on the earth plane is considered a ghost. Many pet-ghosts communicate with the living, often appearing in the same form they occupied when alive, although they usually look more ethereal.

When released fully from the earth plane, an event that can occur anytime after death, a pet's soul often enters one of many heavenly levels of existence, which I call "planes of light." These planes afford many experiences, including rest and restoration, a life review, or the learning of new knowledge, wisdom, and spiritual truths. Once on a plane, a pet might or might not communicate with the living. Sometimes a deceased pet soul is too busy on a heavenly plane to reach back to earth. Some deceased pets become a spiritual guide or teacher for a being that it didn't know during the just-experienced life. And other times, the pet soul can't communicate because it's already starting a new earthly life. Then again, many a pet soul parts the veil and makes contact with former loved ones.

Some pet souls only show up for a certain reason, such as to provide advice or companionship. Others become a spiritual guide. For instance, I once worked with a client who has felt the presence of her cat, Natty, from the time of death onward. Apparently, Natty tells her if a person is nice or not by meowing in different tones. Another client is still connected to a pet ferret that licks her ears, like it did when alive, just for the heck of it.

Sometimes a pet soul appears in a different form when it's dead than it did in the most recent life, much like Kitty did with Granny. I had one client whose pet newt died. A couple of years later, it showed up in a vision looking like the legendary griffin. It told my client that it had once been a griffin and far preferred the griffin form rather than that of a "mere newt."

My former pet guinea pig, Max, also looks different now than when he was alive. Having run the house for nine years, Max's body simply couldn't keep going. He grew a tumor near his shoulder and quickly went downhill. My dogs' veterinarian, who'd heard my stories about Max over the years, euthanized him. I was incredibly sad when I cleaned out Max's cage and gave it away to a neighbor kid. There was only one Max, and I didn't want a replacement guinea pig.

For several weeks the remaining pets, which included two dogs and a cat, were ornery and disorganized. The cat clawed at the dogs, who were shocked at the aberrant treatment. Lucky began hiding my socks behind the couch, spitting his food into the kitchen corners, and pulling other ridiculous pranks. Honey II started scratching out the back screen door. He'd then run out into the backyard, roll in the most offensive and smelly material possible, return to the house, and dirty everything in sight. There was simply no discipline, as General Max had retired.

One day, when wondering how to restore law and order, I felt a presence behind my back. Instinctively, I knew it was Max. Every pet soul has a distinct feeling. But this wasn't the Max I had known. Max's energy felt huge and dispersed, rather like a cloud. I spun around and for a brief moment glimpsed a large white angelic-type figure. I could swear it held a megaphone. The image of "new Max" disappeared as quickly as it appeared, but I knew that Max was back and that he'd be taking charge again.

Almost miraculously, the pets straightened up. Once in a while, I thought I heard a sigh when one of the living pets was particularly foolish. Just like that, they would snap to attention, just like they used to do when Max was alive. Even now I know that Max is still on the job.

How can we best support a pet in finding its right after-death place—and then connecting with it, if we're supposed to? The following exercise will help you release your pet from its body, and the section after the exercise will provide tips for physically and subtly encouraging connection with your deceased pet's soul.

Exercise
Releasing Your Pet with Love

How can you support your dying or already-deceased pet with the transition? We want them to enjoy a smooth journey. The following process can be undertaken no matter what's occurring in your pet's dying, death, or afterlife process.

> **1: Prepare.** Settle into a still place. If your pet is alive, be near it. If it is already deceased, consider holding a memento related to the pet.

> **2: Conduct Spirit-to-Spirit.** Affirm your spirit, your pet's spirit, the helping spirits, and the Spirit.

> **3: Connect to the Pet's Soul.** Ask the Spirit to help you connect with the pet's soul, whether the pet is alive or not. Spend a few moments employing your pet communication skills, which you acquired in chapter 5, and let the soul share how it's doing or feeling. What thoughts are occupying its mind? What feelings is it enjoying or struggling with? Specifically ask the following questions, depending on the state of the soul.
>
> If the pet is alive, ask the pet to reveal which chakra the soul is ensconced in. Are there karmic trappings that, if resolved, would enable the soul to ascend to a higher chakra? Ask the Spirit to assist with this. Could the pet use healing streams to better awaken dharmic truths, fulfill its energetic signature, relieve pain, release attachments, resolve trauma, or deliver messages of love? Is there a wish your pet's soul would like fulfilled; if so, what is it? Send love to your pet's soul and ask the Spirit to bring the soul to whichever chakra or stage in the dying process the Spirit deems best.
>
> If the pet is deceased, no matter how long ago the pet died, request that its soul send you intuitive information about where it is and how it's doing. Is it currently a ghost, hovering on the earth plane? If so, for what reason is it still lingering? Is the soul situated on a plane of light or has it already returned to another earth body? Gather information and ask any questions you have.

You might request to know if the soul still wants to be connected to you, what its presence meant in your life and what you meant to it, or what messages it has for you and other still-living loved ones. Finally, ask the pet's soul and also the Spirit what is best for your pet. Should it remain where it is or be relocated? Healing streams will accompany the soul to the space it needs to occupy.

4: Conclude. Acknowledge that the Spirit will continue supporting your pet and all its loved ones as long as necessary. Send gratitude to your pet and return to your everyday life.

Establishing Afterlife Communication with Your Pet

Once a pet has passed, it might be possible to intuitively communicate with it. I say "possible" because there are several overriding factors, many of which we addressed in this chapter. Yet another barrier can be grief. Sometimes a pet's grief at passing is so severe that its soul needs to process the feelings and memories from its just-lived lifetime before it can communicate. Our own grief can operate like an energetic cloud that prevents connection. Having said that, thousands of my clients receive afterlife communications from their pets, many of which continue or start decades after the pet has passed.

It's helpful to establish the foundation for afterlife communication while your pet is dying, as well as just after its passing. Before the pet dies, conduct Spirit-to-Spirit and ask the Spirit to forge healing streams between your souls. This will help your pet's soul more easily find you after death. You can also request that the Spirit formulate the same bonds between your pet's soul and other household human and nonhuman companions.

Before the death, select and hold a stone or memento when interacting with your pet. This activity will charge the keepsake so you can use it to connect with the deceased pet soul. Previous to or after death, create a small altar. Set this keepsake upon it, as well as others of your pet's beloved objects. You can also review chapter 2. Write (or rewrite) your pet's energetic signature on a slip of paper. Place this note on the altar to remind you of your pet's true nature.

After the pet has died, remain alert. You might sense, feel, or hear your pet. You might see stirrings in the room or spot a depressed place in their bedding. They might also appear in a dream or vision. Frequently, a living pet is more aware of the pet's presence than humans are. If you catch a pet looking around or yapping at "nothing," use your pet communication skills and ask the living pet if they are interacting with their deceased friend. After Honey II died, Lucky, who was a puppy at the time, would pick up one of Honey's favorite toys and toss it across the room. I swear that Honey's spirit threw the ball back.

If you want to more actively cultivate a relationship with a deceased pet, the following steps will make it easier, no matter how much time has passed since your pet's death.

Select a Time Period: Select a specific amount of time during which you'll be available for an outreach from your pet. I recommend choosing between three and seven days. Conduct Spirit-to-Spirit and ask the Spirit to send healing streams to your pet's soul. These streams will invite a visitation. Then pay attention to unusual events. You'll know if they relate to your pet, as your pet will make sure you recognize its message.

Meditate: Set aside a few minutes, hold a pet memento or photograph, and concentrate on your pet. Review its energetic signature and everything your pet meant to you when alive. Then ask the Spirit to help you connect with the pet. Remain open to whatever form the communication takes.

Request a Sign: Conduct Spirit-to-Spirit and ask your pet's soul to send you a sign. You might spy a car with a license plate that features your pet's name or see a billboard that illuminates a special trait of your pet. Your pet will get the message to you!

Share Stories: With your pet's loved ones, share memories aloud about your pet. Talk with the human companions and review special occurrences. You can even speak with the still-living pets. The tales can draw a pet's soul to you and will also assist with the grieving process.

Be open: Above all, be open to however your pet reaches out to you.

Remember, too, this essential truth: love is that bond that never breaks; it only strengthens over time.

Conclusion

Ages ago, members of the nonhuman nations were considered our teachers. They were companions, wayshowers, and friends. Mammals, rodents, birds, reptiles, arthropods, amphibians, aquatic fish…each paid tribute to the Creator and pointed humanity in the right direction. Members of the same family, all beings—human, natural, and even Earth itself—communicated through chakras, subtle energy centers that regulate physical, psychological, and spiritual functions.

Times changed. Natural and human beings were devastated by greed and evil. Fortunately, we are now provided the opportunity to renew the original human/nonhuman bond and transform this earth into a true habitat of love. The key is to care for our pets and cultivate loving pet/human bonds.

Our pets have traveled a great distance to show up in our lives. Like humans, pets have souls. This aspect of a pet, no matter which form it takes, journeys from lifetime to lifetime to work through its blocks to love, thus processing karma, and manifest its spiritual purpose, thereby achieving dharma. Before this lifetime, your pet programmed its karmic objectives and dharmic pursuits into its body. You are key to unlocking your pet's karma and dharma and enabling it to fulfill its objectives. Guess what? Your pet is supporting you in realizing the same goals.

A pet's soul can carry and deposit this vital information because all bodies are equipped with two anatomical systems, each of which processes a distinct type of energy. Energy is information that moves, and it composes everything seen and unseen. The physical anatomy manages physical energy, which is measurable and predictable. Physical energies are governed by the classical laws of science, which make sure that physical reality appears neat and tidy. Subtle energies are ruled by the subtle energy anatomy. Subtle energies, which are also called spiritual, mystical, and psychic energies, are governed by the laws of quantum mechanics, which explain their otherworldly and somewhat miraculous nature. Basically, subtle energies organize physical matter, deciding what will appear or disappear in physical reality, including within your pet.

There are three components of the subtle anatomy. These are the subtle centers, fields, and channels. All three subtle structures can change subtle energy into physical energy and vice versa, thereby serving as energetic transformers. In this book you primarily interacted with your pet's twelve chakras, the main subtle energy centers, toward the goal of converting negative energy into positive energy. The chakras are powerful tools because each stores and regulates specific types of physical, psychological, and spiritual data. They also warehouse a pet's memories, hence they hold the hidden causes of all pet concerns, from trauma to emotional imbalance. With this fact in mind, you acquired several vital concepts and tools aimed at uncovering a pet's causal issues and creating energetic shifts.

Early on, you were taught how to arrive at your pet's energetic signature, its unique set of programs and character traits. You used this data to personalize your subtle energy interactions. The book's main techniques, Spirit-to-Spirit and Healing Streams of Grace, became the basis for all energetic interfaces and also the means for intuitively communicating with your pet and its spiritual guides. And unless you should think that physical activities are useless, you were also shown the benefits of employing vibrational medicines, including essential oils and homeopathy.

In short, all of the material in this book was aimed at fulfilling an age-old obligation: that of creating a more loving relationship between humans and pets. This statement applies to the living pet, but also to the pet that is dying or occupying the afterlife. Overall, every word in this book could actually be considered a gateway to love, for that is the true purpose of the pet/human bond. Because of our pets, we are never alone. Because of us, our pets aren't either.

Resources

Akpan, Nsikan. 2015. "7 Sounds in Nature that Humans Rarely Hear."
PBS Newshour, November 11, 2015.
http://www.pbs.org/newshour/updates/7-sounds-nature
-humans-rarely-hear/.

Aktipis, Athena. 2015. "Hidden Colors: You Can't See Them, But Lizards
Can!" *The Ethogram,* April 6, 2015.
https://theethogram.com/2015/04/06/hidden-colors-you-cant-see
-them-but-lizards-can/.

Altered State. n.d. "Colour Healing."
http://altered-states.net/barry/newsletter220/.

Blake, Stephen, DVM. n.d. "Essential Oil Mini-Guide." *The Pet Whisperer.*
http://www.thepetwhisperer.com/health-tips/oilguide/.

British Homeopathic Association. n.d. "Anxiety."
https://www.britishhomeopathic.org/charity/how-we-can-help
/articles/animals/all-creatures-great-and-small/.

Butler, Ann B., and Rodney M. J. Cotterill. 2006. "Mammalian and Avian
Neuroanatomy and the Question of Consciousness in Birds." *The
Biological Bulletin* 211, no. 2 (October 2006).
http://www.journals.uchicago.edu/doi/full/10.2307/4134586.

Crystalinks, n.d. "Australian Aboriginal Dreamtime."
http://www.crystalinks.com/dreamtime.html.

Crowe, Barbara J. 2004. *Music and Soulmaking.* Lanham, MD: The
Scarecrow Press.

Day, Christopher. 2002. "Homeopathy for Cage and Aviary Birds." *Holistic Bird Newsletter*, Summer 2002. https://holisticbirdnewsletter.wordpress.com/modalities /homeopathy-for-cage-and-aviary-birds/.

Dodero Hearing Center. 2013. "How Do Cockroaches, Cats, and Other Species Hear?" February 2013. http://www.doderohearing.com/blog/how-do-cockroaches-cats -and-other-species-hear/.

Dvorsky, George. 2013. "Brain Scans Show That Dogs Are as Conscious as Human Children." October 7, 2013. https://io9.gizmodo.com/brain-scans-show-that-dogs -are-as-conscious-as-human-ch-1442003302.

Goodnet. 2015. "5 Animals with Incredible Healing Powers." January 9, 2015. http://www.goodnet.org/articles/5-animals -incredible-healing-powers-list.

Graham, Lynne, et al. 2005. "The Influence of Olfactory Stimulation on the Behaviour of Dogs Housed in a Rescue Shelter." *Applied Animal Behaviour Science* 01 (2005): 143–153. http://www.appliedanimalbehaviour.com/article /S0168-1591%2804%2900197-2/abstract.

Grantham, Bill. n.d. *Creation Myths and Legends of the Creek Indians.* Gainseville, FL: The University Press of Florida, 2002. http:// ufdcimages.uflib.ufl.edu/AA/00/01/16/79/00001 /CreationMythsofCreekIndians.pdf.

Habacher, G., et al. 2006. "Effectiveness of Acupuncture in Veterinary Medicine: Systematic Review." *Journal of Veterinarian Internal Medicine* (2006): 480–486. https://www.ncbi.nlm.nih.gov/pubmed/16734078.

Haekel, Josef. n.d. "Totemism." *Encyclopaedia Britannica.* https://www.britannica.com/topic/totemism-religion.

Hadhazy, Adam. 2010. "Think Twice: How the 'Gut Brain' Influences Mood and Well-Being." *Scientific American*, February 12, 2010. https://www.scientificamerican.com/article/gut-second-brain/.

Heimbuch, Jaymi. 2016. "6 Medical Conditions That Dogs Can Sniff Out." *Mother Nature Network*, June 28, 2016. https://www.mnn.com/family/pets/stories/6-medical-conditions-that-dogs-can-sniff.

Hubbard, Sylvia Booth. 2015. "What Your Pet Says About Your Personality." *Newsmax*, November 13, 2015. http://www.newsmax.com/Health/Headline/pet-personality-traits-owner/2015/11/13/id/702033/.

Hunt, Valerie V., et al. n.d. "A Study of Structural Integration from Neuromuscular, Energy Field, and Emotional Approaches." http://rolfing-ca.com/PDF/ucla.pdf.

IABC, n.d. "International Association for Biologically Closed Electric Circuits (BCEC) in Medicine and Biology." http://www.iabc.readywebsites.com/page/page/623957.htm.

Lee Foundation, n.d. "The Rife Microscope or 'Facts and Their Fate.'" Reprint No. 25A. Lee Foundation for Nutritional Research, Milwaukee, WI.

Link, John. 2007. "What Percentage of the Electromagnetic Spectrum Is Visible Light?" *MadSci Network: Physics*, August 27, 2007. http://www.madsci.org/posts/archives/2007-08/1188407794.Ph.r.html.

Lucas, Stephanie. 2014. "How Ancient Cultures Used Healing Crystals and Stones." November 9, 2014. https://quantumstones.com/ancient-cultures-used-healing-crystals-stones/.

Lyons, Leslie A. 2003. "Why Do Cats Purr?" *Scientific American*, January 27, 2003. https://www.scientificamerican.com/article/why-do-cats-purr/.

Main, Bevan S., et al. 2017. "Microbial Immuno-Communication in Neurodegenerative Diseases." *Frontiers in Neuroscience*, March 23, 2017. https://www.ncbi.nlm.nih.gov/pmc/articles/PMC5362619/.

McCraty, Rolin, PhD, et al. 2015. "The Heart Has Its Own 'Brain' and Consciousness." *In5d*, January 10, 2015. http://in5d.com/the-heart-has-its-own-brain-and-consciousness/.

Mom.me. n.d. "What Mammals Make Sounds That Humans Cannot Hear?" http://animals.mom.me/mammal-sounds-humans-cannot-hear-5615.html.

Natural Connections Healthcare. n.d. "Björn Nordenström: Biologically Closed Electric Circuits and Other Important Information on Microcurrents." http://www.naturalworldhealing.com/nordenstrom-electrical.htm.

Pappas, Stephanie. 2016. "There Might be 1 Trillion Species on Earth." *Livescience*, May 5, 2016. https://www.livescience.com/54660-1-trillion-species-on-earth.html.

Pet Health Council. n.d. "Benefits of Owning a Pet." http://www.hopeforpets.org/Benefits%20of%20Owning%20a%20Pet.htm.

Peterson, Paula. n.d. "The Cat's Purr and Other Sounds that Heal." *Earthcode*. http://paulapeterson.com/CatsPurr.html.

The Rescue Animal MP3 Project. n.d. "Music Studies." http://rescueanimalmp3.org/music-studies/.

Rexresearch.com. n.d. "Björn Nordenström." http://www.rexresearch.com/nordenstrom/nordenstrom.htm.

Rovner, Julie. 2012. "Pet Therapy: How Animals and Humans Heal Each Other." *Shots/MPR*, March 5, 2012. http://www.npr.org/sections/health-shots/2012/03/09/146583986/pet-therapy-how-animals-and-humans-heal-each-other.

Sanders, Laura. 2016. "Microbes Can Play Games with the Mind."
ScienceNews, March 23, 2016.
https://www.sciencenews.org/article/microbes-can
-play-games-mind.

Scott, Dana. n.d. "Essential Oils for Dogs." *Dogsnaturally*.
http://www.dogsnaturallymagazine.com/essential-oils-for-dogs/.

Shelton, Melissa. 2012. *The Animal Desk Reference: Essential Oils for
Animals*. CreateSpace: April 15, 2012.

Volk, Jeff. n.d. "Shaping Up with Sound."
http://www.cymaticsource.com/pdf/ks_shaping%20up_06.pdf.

Walker, Kaetheryn. 1998. *Homeopathic First Aid*. Rochester, VT: Healing
Arts Press.

Wagner, Kathryn Drury. 2013. "The Science Behind Healing
with Sound." *Spirituality & Health*, December 16, 2013.
https://spiritualityhealth.com/articles/2013/12/16/
science-behind-healing-sound.

Walker, Pete. n.d. "The Four F's: A Trauma Typology in Complex
PTSD."
http://pete-walker.com/fourFs_TraumaTypologyComplexPTSD.
htm.

Waters, Frank. 1963. *The Book of Hopi*. New York: Ballantine Books.

Whistler Veterinarian Clinic. n.d. "Homeopathy."
http://www.whistlervetservices.ca/homeopathic-first-aid-for-pets/.

Wolchover, Natalie. 2012. "What Type of Music Do Pets Like?"
Livescience, March 19, 2012.
https://www.livescience.com/33780-animal-music-pets.html.

Wonderopolis. n.d. "How Can Dogs Hear Things We Can't?" Life
Science.
https://wonderopolis.org/wonder/how-can-dogs-hear-things
-we-cant-2.

Yu, Chuan. 1995. *Traditional Chinese Veterinary Acupuncture and Moxibustion*. Chinese Agricultural Press. Ebook edition available from China Scientific Books at https://www.chinascientificbooks .com/traditional-chinese-veterinary-acupuncture-and -moxibustionebook-p-87/.

GET MORE AT LLEWELLYN.COM

Visit us online to browse hundreds of our books and decks, plus sign up to receive our e-newsletters and exclusive online offers.

- Free tarot readings • Spell-a-Day • Moon phases
- Recipes, spells, and tips • Blogs • Encyclopedia
- Author interviews, articles, and upcoming events

GET SOCIAL WITH LLEWELLYN

Find us on 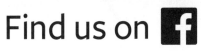 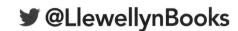 @LlewellynBooks

www.Facebook.com/LlewellynBooks

GET BOOKS AT LLEWELLYN

LLEWELLYN ORDERING INFORMATION

 Order online: Visit our website at www.llewellyn.com to select your books and place an order on our secure server.

 Order by phone:
- Call toll free within the US at 1-877-NEW-WRLD (1-877-639-9753)
- We accept VISA, MasterCard, American Express, and Discover.
- Canadian customers must use credit cards.

 Order by mail:
Send the full price of your order (MN residents add 6.875% sales tax) in US funds plus postage and handling to: Llewellyn Worldwide, 2143 Wooddale Drive, Woodbury, MN 55125-2989

POSTAGE AND HANDLING

STANDARD (US):
(Please allow 12 business days)
$30.00 and under, add $6.00.
$30.01 and over, FREE SHIPPING.

INTERNATIONAL ORDERS,
INCLUDING CANADA:
$16.00 for one book, plus $3.00 for each additional book.

Visit us online for more shipping options. Prices subject to change.

FREE CATALOG!

To order, call
1-877-
NEW-WRLD
ext. 8236
or visit our
website

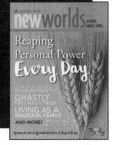

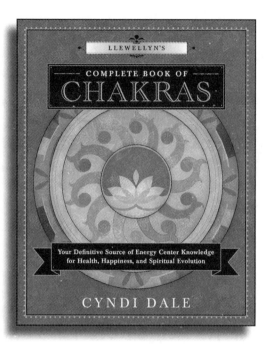

LLEWELLYN'S

COMPLETE BOOK OF

CHAKRAS

Your Definitive Source of Energy Center Knowledge
for Health, Happiness, and Spiritual Evolution

CYNDI DALE

Llewellyn's Complete Book of Chakras

Your Definitive Source of Energy Center Knowledge for Health, Happiness, and Spiritual Evolution

Cyndi Dale

As powerful centers of subtle energy, the chakras have fascinated humanity for thousands of years. *Llewellyn's Complete Book of Chakras* is a unique and empowering resource that provides comprehensive insights into these foundational sources of vitality and strength. Discover what chakras and chakra systems are, how to work with them for personal growth and healing, and the ways our understanding of chakras has transformed throughout time and across cultures.

Lively and accessible, this definitive reference explores the science, history, practices, and structures of our subtle energy. With an abundance of illustrations and a wealth of practical exercises, Cyndi Dale shows you how to use chakras for improving wellness, attracting what you need, obtaining guidance, and expanding your consciousness.

978-0-7387-3962-5
8 x 10 · 1,056 pp. · $39.99

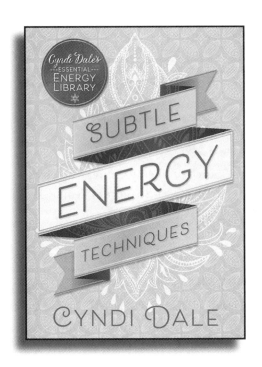

SUBTLE

ENERGY

TECHNIQUES

CYNDI DALE

Subtle Energy Techniques
Book 1 of Cyndi Dale's
Essential Energy Library

Cyndi Dale

Renowned author Cyndi Dale invites you into the world of subtle energy, where you'll explore auras, chakras, intuition, and the basics of her groundbreaking energy techniques. Whether your goals are physical, psychological, or spiritual, these methods can help you achieve your desires, heal your wounds, and live an enlightened life.

978-0-7387-5161-0
5 x 7 · 288 pp. · $14.99

· · · · · · · · · · · · · · · ·

To Write to the Author

If you wish to contact the author or would like more information about this book, please write to the author in care of Llewellyn Worldwide Ltd. and we will forward your request. Both the author and the publisher appreciate hearing from you and learning of your enjoyment of this book and how it has helped you. Llewellyn Worldwide Ltd. cannot guarantee that every letter written to the author can be answered, but all will be forwarded.

Please write to:

Cyndi Dale
℅ Llewellyn Worldwide
2143 Wooddale Drive
Woodbury, MN 55125-2989

Please enclose a self-addressed stamped envelope for reply or $1.00 to cover costs. If outside the USA, enclose an international postal reply coupon.

Many of Llewellyn's authors have websites with additional information and resources. For more information, please visit our website at

WWW.LLEWELLYN.COM